MW00905471

The Cure of Chronic Hepatitis B
One Man's Cure
One Family's Experience

Kunmi and Ibiyinka Oluleye

IROK Solutions, Inc.
Cambridge, Massachusetts
1996

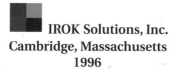

The Cure of Chronic Hepatitis B
One Man's Cure
One Family's Experience

By Kunmi and Ibiyinka Oluleye

Published by:

IROK Solutions Inc.
1770 Mass Avenue, Suite 134
Cambridge, MA 02140 U.S.A.

Oluleye, Kunmi.
The cure of chronic hepatitis B: one man's cure, one family's experience / by Kunmi and Ibiyinka Oluleye.
p. cm.
Includes index.
Preassigned LCCN: 96-94867
ISBN 0-9654801-9-4

1. Hepatitis B--Patients--Biography. I. Oluleye, Ibiyinka II. Title.

RC848.H44O68 1997 616.3'623'09
QBI96-40496

Printed in the United States of America

CONTENTS

FOREWORD

Hepatitis B and C causes liver cancer, the number one cause of cancer deaths worldwide. Hepatitis B causes liver cancer fifty percent of the time, while Hepatitis C causes liver cancer the other fifty percent of the time.

There are more than 350 million people in the world who are infected with Chronic Hepatitis B. 0.1 to 0.5 of that are in the United States and Western Europe. However, up to five to twenty percent has been found in the Far East and in some tropical countries. As high as thirty percent in persons with Down Syndrome, leprosy, leukemia and Hodgkin's disease.[1] More and more hospitals are vaccinating babies at birth against these deadly disease.

In 1994, my husband was diagnosed with Chronic Hepatitis B. In 1995, he underwent a revolutionary combination treatment with Ribavirin and Interferon Alfa-2b and was cured. *The medical community prefers to use the term "virus negative."* He is probably the first, in the United States to undergo this combination treatment.

There is no single source of detailed advice which helps the infected victim to cope and hopefully cure the disease, so we decided to write one.

As a career woman, a mother and wife whose husband was infected with Chronic Hepatitis B virus and cured, I felt the need for such information and the universal appeal a book would have on this subject. We have first hand experience with every aspect of this devastating disease, including the revolutionary treatment of Interferon Alfa-2b and Ribavirin, which has proven effective. My story, that of my husband's is a riveting account of modern medicine, human emotion, urban pressure and very basic nutritional intake and health care.

This book is a great resource for anyone associated with hepatitis directly or indirectly. Every hepatologist, victim, family or friend of the victim, nurse, medical student, everyone.

Reference:

1. Wilson, Braunwald, Isselbacher, Petersdorf, Martin, Fauci and Root. *Harrison's Principles of Internal Medicine,* p. 1327.

ACKNOWLEDGEMENTS

Thanks go first to God for giving Ibi the confidence to undergo this treatment, and for keeping me sane during the ordeal.

I would like to thank Dr. Najarian for the important medical information contained in Chapter Three and having the vision to suggest and administer the combination treatment.

Thanks goes to Yemisi Oluwole, Kemi and Mabayoje Tuyo, Dean Elizabeth Rawlins, Ms. Veronica Folayan, Carla Ulebor and Jane Nash of Simmons GSM Library for reviewing the book.

Thanks to the Oluleye Family, especially Daddy, the Major General, late Mrs. Olajumoke Oluleye whom we believe was with us in spirit, Dr. Wole and Layemi; my Aunt and Uncle, Mr. and Mrs. Tuyo of Houston, Texas, for their love and support prior to, during and after the treatment.

Finally thanks to Ms. Roberta Green for always being there and being the best friend anyone could ask for. She was not only an inspiration, but truly someone to lean on whenever needed and as many times as necessary.

Warning - Disclaimer

This book provides information about our experience with Chronic Hepatitis B and the combination treatment that cured the disease. It is sold with the understanding that the publisher and authors are not engaged in rendering medical services. If medical or other expert assistance is required, the services of a competent doctor or professional should be sought.

Every effort has been made to make this book as complete and as accurate as possible. However, there may be mistakes both typographical and in content. Therefore, this text should be used only as a general guide and not as the ultimate source of treating Hepatitis B.

The authors and IROK Solutions, Inc. shall have neither liability nor responsibility to any person or entity for any loss or damage caused, or alleged to be caused, directly or indirectly by the information contained in this book.

If you do not wish to be bound by the above, you may return this book to the publisher for a full refund.

Chapter One

Take control of your life.

Meet the Patient and His Family

Ibiyinka (Ibi for short) was born and raised in Nigeria. He is a Northeastern University graduate who at the time of the Hepatitis treatment, worked as an Environmental Health and Safety Specialist for a University in Boston. He now works with software in the computer industry. When Dr. Najarian diagnosed him with Hepatitis B, Ibi was unsure as to how he became infected.

My name is Kunmi and I am your narrator. I was also born and raised in Nigeria. I finished high school and graduate studies in the United States.

Ibi and I kept separate diaries and promised to not read the other's entries until after the treatment. All entries shown here are with minor editing.

The journal entries in this chapter were written prior to the beginning of the treatment.

PERSONAL DOCUMENTATION OF THE DISCOVERY OF HEPATITIS B AND DECISION TO ACCEPT THE ALTERNATIVE COMBINATION TREATMENT

Ibi's Journal

On October 19, 1994, I called my insurance company for a referral to a doctor. That morning, I experienced cold and fever-like symptoms. Since I lived in Belmont, Massachusetts, I was given the name of a doctor in the same town. His name was Dr. Thomas Najarian. The name sounded native to the country that I am from, Nigeria, but he is Armenian. I called the doctor and he said he would like to see me as soon as possible. I made an appointment to see him sometime that afternoon. He performed a physical and took my blood for testing. The test for strep throat was negative. He prescribed some antibiotics for my symptoms.

I could see that he was sympathetic to my needs because he paid close attention to me and wanted to know all about my health. For my blood test, he requested a test for the Hepatitis B Virus (HBV), white blood count and liver function test.

A few days later, the results of my blood test came back and the doctor called me, saying he would like to repeat the tests to confirm the results. He patiently explained the results of the tests to me. He told me my HBV vaccine level was not noticeable, and that my liver enzymes were higher than normal. I told him my previous doctor knew about the liver enzymes, but told me there was nothing to worry about and gave me the Hepatitis vaccine. Dr. Najarian then asked me if I had been tested for HBV before I got the vaccine. I told him no. I assumed that my previous doctor must have done that. Dr. Najarian then requested I have my medical report sent to him from the Harvard Community doctor. He told me that a high percentage of people from Africa have this virus and that he was going to repeat the test.

I was a little scared because he told me he thought

I had HBV, and he mentioned that there was no cure for the virus. He said some people had been cured with Interferon Alpha but there was a forty percent chance of cure, and over time, there was remission. He later alluded to a combination therapy that had been used in Europe. In this therapy, Ribavirin and Interferon Alpha were used. He then said the Ribavirin medicine was not yet approved by the United States Food and Drug Administration. He said the combination therapy had an eighty percent cure rate. That reinforced my hope of a possible cure, if the repeated tests were found to be positive.

Dr. Najarian continued by saying if I would like the treatment, I could get the Ribavirin from any pharmacy in Mexico. He did not know the cost of the medication. He also said that HBV takes years before it makes one sick.

He took his time explaining my chances and alternatives for cure. Another blood test for white count, liver function, and HBV surface antigens were done. It was POSITIVE!! He requested at the time that everyone around me should take the HBV vaccine. My fiancée, Kunmi, and son, Sayo had to be vaccinated against HBV.

Dr. Najarian asked for a face-to-face discussion with me in December, 1994, focusing on which treatment I would like to pursue. It was obvious that he had done a lot of research on Hepatitis B, C and E. He told me that he had called some doctors in Europe to find out more about the treatments available for the virus. He furnished me with a lot of information about HBV. He even made copies of journals and medical books for me to read. I was well informed about my alternatives and chances.

Kunmi and I sought other opinions about the combination treatment from doctors at Massachusetts General Hospital. The head of the Hepatology Department and his next in command discouraged me from undergoing such a treatment. They urged me to participate in their studies, which would be at no cost to me. At this point I was frustrated and worried about my health. I started to pray very hard for God to help me make the best decision. I went with my instincts because that was all that I had left to rely on.

I made up my mind and was determined to undergo the combination therapy of Ribavirin and Interferon Alpha. Dr. Najarian informed me fully about documented side effects of the combination treatment. He was unsure of how I would react to this treatment, and he wanted me to really think through my decision before going ahead with the combination treatment. I told him that I had decided to undergo the treatment because the attack process of the drugs on the virus made sense. I knew if I stayed on the treatment I would be cured. The attack process of the drug is that it weakens the virus. The more drug one takes the weaker the virus gets. As the virus attempts to mutate itself to one drug, the other drug weakens it. The virus cannot fight both drugs at once, therefore, it weakens to the point of destruction.

The journey to Mexico began. I flew to Houston with my fiancée and her son for the holidays. Two days after Christmas, we headed for Laredo in Mexico to buy the Ribavirin. It was a sixteen-hour drive to and from. When we arrived we started looking around for pharmacies. The pharmacy names where written in Spanish. Every word we came across was written in Spanish. None of us knew how to read Spanish but putting two and two together we came up with some meanings for the Spanish words. The first pharmacy we went to had only one box with twelve capsules of 200 mg of Ribavirin. We needed to buy 1,200 capsules of 200 mg each. We went to another pharmacy, and they only had two boxes of 400 mg of Ribavirin. I started getting concerned that I might not find enough medication for my treatment. We went to another store and we were told that they could get us fifteen boxes of 400 mg of Ribavirin. There were twelve capsules in each box, meaning they had a total of 180 capsules.

At this point cost was no longer an issue for me. I just wanted to find enough medication to buy for my treatment. There was another store down the road and it seemed to be the last pharmacy in sight. To our surprise they had the exact dosage of Ribavirin that we were looking for, and the cost was even cheaper than the fifteen boxes we had requested from the previous pharmacy. We bought more packages than necessary because I did not want to get to Boston and find out that I needed more. What if the dosage necessary for the cure was more than projected? Besides, Dr. Najarian said he would buy all the leftover drugs from me. It was a nice gesture on his part.

After buying the Ribavirin, I was concerned about getting it through the border into the United States. Dr. Najarian gave me a note to show the authorities prior to going to Houston, stating that the Ribavirin was for my personal use, for the cure of Hepatitis B. He added that if I had any problems, I should call him. We bought sombreros, blankets and other souvenirs and placed the Ribavirin in the same bag.

We were asked at the border if we were citizens. I said I was not and handed over my green card for verification. We were told to go on without hassle.

On December 29, 1994, we left Houston. I called my doctor the following day, and we scheduled an appointment to perform other tests before starting the treatment. He promised me he would do everything in his power to make sure I got well. This promise gave me confidence that he had my welfare at heart.

When I saw Dr. Najarian in January 1995, he took more blood for testing. He tested for the HBV surface antigen, e-antigen, WBC, and a liver function test. All the antigen tests came out positive and my white blood count (WBC) was below normal. He mentioned that he would see me every week until he felt comfortable that I was doing fine. Treatment began on January 18, 1995 and ended June 21st, 1995.

Kunmi's Journal

I was shocked when Ibi told me that he had Hepatitis B. First, I did not know what it was. Secondly, after I understood what it was, how did he get it? I kept saying, "Are you sure?" I insisted on a second, third and fourth opinion. At the end of the day, yes he had it. Why didn't the Harvard Community doctor detect it? If Dr. Najarian had not noticed it, Ibi could have suffered permanent liver damage and/or died.

I went to all of Ibi's meetings with Dr. Najarian, in which he educated us about the alternatives, including the combination treatment of Ribavirin and Interferon. I was extremely skeptical. How can I trust this doctor? Does he know what he is doing? My skepticism must have shown through. I asked a lot of questions and the doctor seemed intimidated, but he explained his points calmly.

Before we went to Mexico to purchase the Ribavirin, Dr. Najarian videotaped the final meeting with himself, Ibi and me. He also had us sign a release confirming that Ibi had been properly informed of the side effects of his treatment with Interferon Alfa and Ribavirin.

I was terrified by the side effects of the treatment. Fevers, headaches, body aches and extreme depression that could lead to suicide were common. Ibi made a decision which I didn't like, but had to support. While on the phone to Ibi's family in Nigeria, I informed his father and oldest brother of his condition, and his decision to undergo this combination treatment. His oldest brother asked me to spell Ribavirin and Interferon Alfa. Our guess it that out of concern, they wanted to double check the proper use of the drugs with their Nigerian family doctor. A few weeks later during another conversation, they were deeply concerned.

I made sure they understood this was Ibi's sole decision and that I had to and would support him. I felt sure that I communicated to them what lay ahead of us. I asked for their emotional support and that they call us and speak to Ibi often.

If he was depressed and could not discuss it with

discuss it with me, there were four male family members he could turn to.

I asked for moral support from my family. I called my Aunt, Mrs. Harriet Tuyo, a nurse practitioner in Houston. She was extremely helpful in helping me understand the medical terminology. She too asked a lot of questions, which I then asked the doctor. By December 1994, I was mentally and emotionally ready to take on this beast called Hepatitis B.

There remained the matter of whether or not to tell my son, Sayo. He was five years old and had enough trouble understanding why I wouldn't let him buy a toy, or go to McDonalds or Burger King. Since he and Ibi spent a great deal of time together, due to my hectic schedule, I needed to prepare him for what lay ahead. I talked with him in a roundabout way about people being sick and the need to be nice and less demanding of them. I then told him that supposing I was sick, I would like him to be on his best behavior and ask Daddy for things more than me. I then explained that when he got sick, I didn't ask him to do his chores.

One weekend when he was in a great mood, I told him that Daddy would be taking some medicine for a long time that would make him sick, and we needed to be nice to him. He said okay. I also explained that Daddy might be more quiet and cranky because of the medicine.

I told him that he and I would have to get three shots each to help us not get the disease because we lived with Daddy. He did not take the idea of getting shots too well, so I offered him a deal of one dollar for every shot he got. He agreed, but there was a concerned look on his face. We were both quiet.

Some time passed and he asked if Daddy was going to die. I told him he would not. He asked me if I were sure, and I reassured him that I was. I told him that he could come to Daddy's appointment with us if he wanted, and he did. He asked the doctor a similar question. Dr. Najarian was excellent in his answer. He told Sayo that Ibi would be taking some medicine that might make him a little different for a little while but that there was nothing to worry about.

I made arrangements to have Sayo and me vaccinated for Hepatitis. The vaccination was three shots over a six month period. Sayo got his first shot in November, 1994 and the last one in May, 1995. Mine began later, and I am yet to get the third shot.

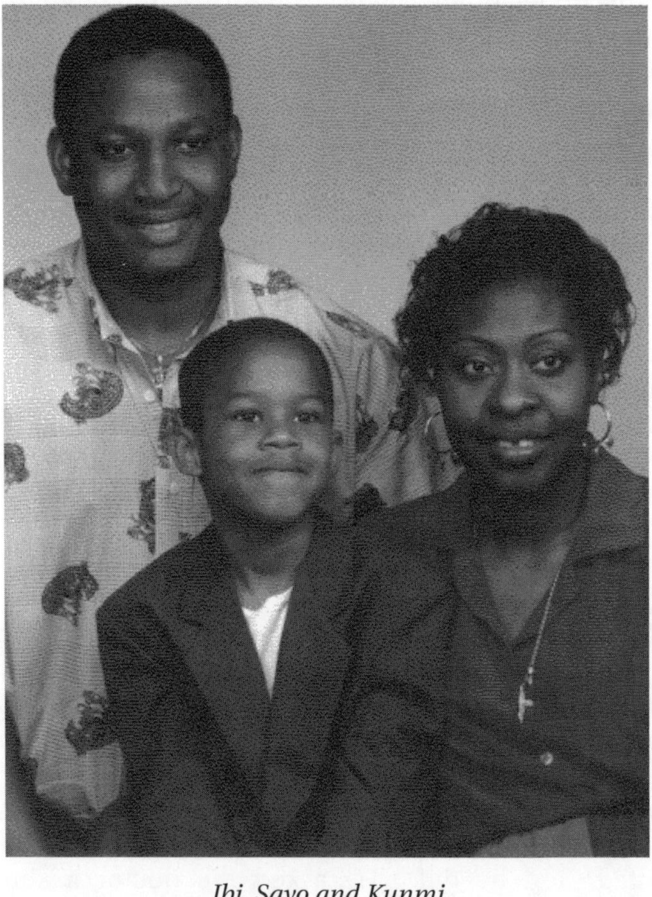

Ibi, Sayo and Kunmi

Chapter Two

Knowledge is power.

What is Hepatitis?

Hepatitis A — Formerly called **"Infectious Hepatitis."** This is most common in children in developing countries but is seen frequently in adults in the western world. It is spread through contaminated food and water.

Hepatitis B — Formerly called **"Serum Hepatitis."** This is the most serious form of Hepatitis, with 350 million carriers in the world and an estimated one million carriers in the United States. Each year, there are approximately 200,000 new cases in the United States. An estimated 17,000-20,000 pregnant women are carriers of the Hepatitis B virus and can pass the infection on to their newborn babies at the time of delivery and possibly also to their sexual partner(s). Chronic Hepatitis B causes liver cirrhosis or cancer, the number one cause of cancer deaths worldwide, fifty percent of the time.

Hepatitis C — Formerly called **"Non-A/Non-B Hepatitis."** It has infected 3.5 million people in the United States, of which 26,000 die each year. Hepatitis C causes liver cirrhosis or cancer, the number one cause of cancer deaths worldwide, the other fifty percent of the time.

Hepatitis D — Formerly called **"Delta Hepatitis."** This form is found mainly in intravenous drug users who are carriers of the Hepatitis B virus. Being a carrier is a requirement for the necessary Hepatitis D virus to develop and spread.

Hepatitis E — Formerly called **"Enteric or Epidemic Non-A, Non-B Hepatitis."** It's commonly found in the Indian Ocean and spread through fecal-oral routes.

Hepatitis D and E are rare in the United States. Infection within the family can occur with Hepatitis A, B, C or E. Prompt diagnosis and appropriate precautions with immune shots called Gamma Globulin or vaccination are important for those who are exposed.

Adequate sanitation and good personal hygiene will reduce the spread of Hepatitis A and E. Water should be boiled prior to its use if any question of safety exists. Similarly, in areas where sanitation is questionable, food should be cooked well and fruits peeled. Those planning to travel to areas where Hepatitis A is widespread are advised to take Hepatitis A vaccine before leaving. Dentists, doctors, nurses, laboratory technicians, and others who may draw blood, perform surgical procedures or handle sharp instruments must be informed that the virus is present so that adequate precautions can be taken.

Hepatitis is known as the alphabet disease because there's also Hepatitis F and G. Limited information is availabe at this time.

Questions and Answers About Hepatitis B

What is Hepatitis B?

Hepatitis B is an infection of the liver caused by the Hepatitis B virus (HBV). The virus is found in bodily fluids, including semen, saliva, blood and urine.

About one-third of the people with HBV have a completely "silent" disease. The term "silent" means that even though the disease is present, there are no symptoms. When symptoms are present, they may be mild or severe. They include fever, headaches, muscle aches, fatigue, loss of appetite, vomiting and diarrhea. Later stages may be marked by dark urine, abdominal pain and yellowing of the skin and the whites of the eyes (NIAID, 1992).

Some people recover from Hepatitis B within several weeks and develop antibodies (protectants) from HBV. However five to ten percent of people infected never develop antibodies and may harbor the virus for many years or their entire lives. Chronic carriers, as they are referred to, may have very few symptoms and may not be aware that they have the virus. Others have ongoing liver problems resulting in persistent Hepatitis, liver failure or liver cancer.

What is the connection between mental retardation and Hepatitis B?

Hepatitis B is found most frequently among people who live in congregate housing situations, such as group homes, institutions and nursing homes. People who work with these residents are also at risk of infection.

People with Down's Syndrome are more susceptible to Hepatitis B (HBV) infection. For unknown reasons, their immune systems respond differently to the presence of HBV. It is also documented that they are at an increased risk of catching and of being carriers of Hepatitis B.

Who is at risk for Hepatitis B?

Anyone can get Hepatitis B; however certain populations have especially high rates of infection. These include health care workers, Asians and Pacific Islanders, Haitians, Sub-Saharan Africans, Alaskan Eskimos, persons with multiple sex partners who do not practice safe sex, and institutionalized populations (AAPCHO, 1992).

Does Hepatitis B affect fertility?

No it does not. Women who are infected can still get pregnant and infected men can still impregnate women.

How is Hepatitis B spread?

Hepatitis B can be spread unknowingly in several different ways:

** Contact with infected blood or bodily fluids containing blood, such as semen, vaginal/menstrual fluids, tears, saliva, breast milk or urine. Infection may then occur through scratches, cuts, bites, rashes, mouth-to-mouth contact, sexual activity, kissing or biting.

** HBV can also be spread through contact with contaminated syringes, razors, or other objects containing infected human blood. Processes that would use such objects include tatoos, electrolysis and acupunture.

** Pregnant women who have the Hepatitis B virus can pass it to their babies, usually during the birth process. Vaccination at birth, with additional shots at one/two and six months of age can prevent Hepatitis B in these children.

How can Hepatitis B be diagnosed?

The only sure way to diagnose Hepatitis B is by testing blood for HBV. Blood tests can confirm HBV infection, as well as identify carriers most likely to transmit the disease to others.

Evidence of Hepatitis B infection is shown by the presence in the blood of Hepatitis B surface antigen and Hepatitis B e-antigen.

How is Hepatitis B treated prior to the combination therapy?

Interferon Alfa-2b is effective in the treatment of adults who have Chronic Hepatitis B virus infection. The recommended dose of Interferon Alfa-2b for the treatment of Chronic Hepatitis B is 5,000,000 units daily, administered by subcutaneous or intramuscular injec-tion, for a total of sixteen weeks. The patient must be monitored carefully during the treatment period for side effects including flu-like symptoms, depression, rashes, abnormal blood counts and other reactions.

A recently published meta-analysis of several randomized trials of Interferon Alfa-2b in the treatment of patients with Chronic Hepatitis B showed such treatment to be cost-effective (Wong et al. Annals Intern. Med. 1995; 122:664-675). This analysis showed that treatment with Interferon Alfa-2b decreased viral replication, documented by loss of serum Hepatitis B e-antigen, in about forty-five percent of patients compared to less than ten percent of untreated patients. About eight percent of patients also lost Hepatitis B virus surface antigen (completely cured) within one year of treatment compared to a rate of about one percent year for untreated patients.

Interferon Alfa-2b treatment of Chronic Hepatitis B requires careful medical attention. One should contact a doctor for more information.

What is the combination treatment?

The combination treatment is the use of Interferon Alfa-2b with Ribavirin (also known as Virazole). There is growing interest within the medical community about using Ribavirin and Interferon Alfa in a combination treatment. The combination is more effective than either drug alone without increased toxicity.

Schering Plough Corporation is the pharmaceutical company in the United States that manufactures Interferon Alfa-2b. ICN Pharmaceutical is the manufacturer of Ribavirin. In Mexico, Ribavirin is approved for seven diseases: Herpes Simplex Virus (HSV), Respiratory Syncytial Virus (RSV), Hepatitis, Influenza, Varicella Zoster Virus (VZV), Chicken Pox and Measles.

Interferon Alfa-2b administered by intramuscular or subcutaneous injection is indicated for the treatment of Chronic Hepatitis B and Chronic Hepatitis C. Interferon Alfa is a naturally occurring glycoprotein that is secreted by cells in response to viral infections. It exerts its effects by binding to a membrane receptor. Receptor binding leads to enhanced expression of certain genes. This further leads to the enhancement and induction of certain cellular activities, including augmentation of target cell killing by lymphocytes and inhibition of virus replication in infected cells.

Side effects caused by Interferon treatment are frequent "flu-like" symptoms, depression, headache, and decreased appetite. The flu-like symptoms can be minimized by taking two doses of acetaminophen, for example, Tylenol. In addition, Interferon may depress the bone marrow leading to difficulties with white blood cells and platelets.

Ribavirin is in capsules of 200mg and 400mg. It can cause reversible hemolytic anemia.

The combination treatment for Chronic Hepatitis B discussed in this book is an alternative for those infected.

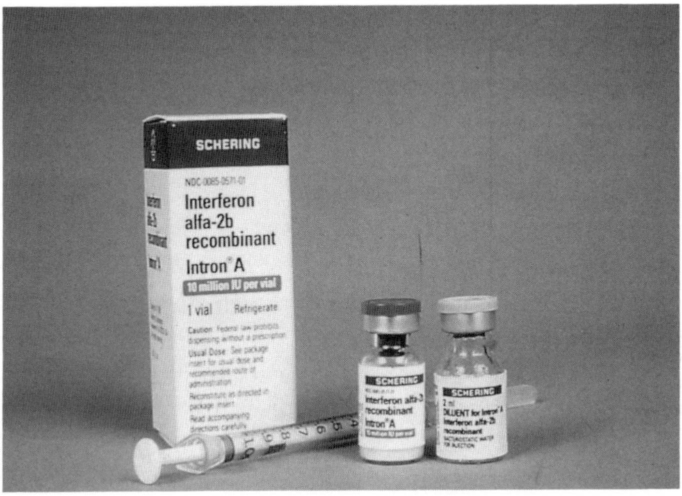

Interferon Alfa-2b

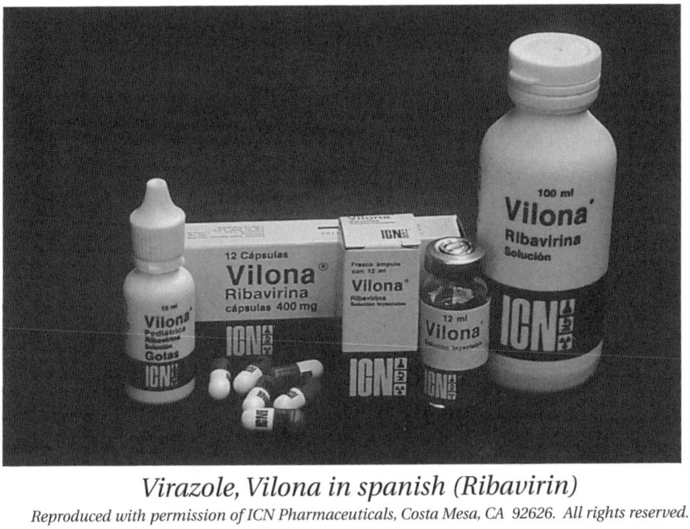

Virazole, Vilona in spanish (Ribavirin)

What other factors help the treatment?

While undergoing treatment, patients should:

- avoid exertion
- eat a balanced, low fat diet
- avoid alcohol and smoking
- use medications only when advised by a doctor (AAPCHO, 1992).

How can Hepatitis B be prevented?

People who have never been exposed to the Hepatitis B virus may be protected through vaccination. In 1991, the Immunization Practices Advisory Committee of the Public Health Service recommended that all children be vaccinated. The Centers for Disease Control and Prevention estimates that from 200,000 to 300,000 cases occur annually because adults have been reluctant to get the vaccine that has been on the market for over ten years. If all children receive the vaccine, eventually Hepatitis B will be eliminated.

The vaccine is especially recommended for:

- healthcare workers
- household members of a person with Chronic Hepatitis
- newborn children of mothers with HBV
- staff in residences for people with mental retardation and Hepatitis.

In order for pregnant women to avoid passing HBV to their newborns, all pregnant women should be tested. This will determine if they are silent carriers of the disease. If they are, their infant can be vaccinated.

How can Hepatitis B be prevented when the infected person lives in the home?

Handwashing is the single most important hygiene practice that can reduce the chance of infected blood or contaminated fluids being transmitted. Careful handwashing with soap and water should be used:

- when caring for bleeding wounds
- when handling items which have been contaminated with blood
- after each bathroom use
- before eating

Household members should avoid sharing personal items that may have traces of blood or body secretions, such as razors, clippers, toothbrushes, eating utensils and hypodermic needles.

Efforts should also be made to reduce the possibility of blood contact. Bleeding or oozing cuts should be covered. People doing the cleaning should protect themselves by wearing disposable gloves, especially when discarding soiled materials. If anything becomes contaminated with blood from a carrier, clean immediately with household bleach, soap and water.

The information in this chapter is a merge of data from various sources. Each source had slightly different explanations of hepatitis, symptoms and numbers of people infected.

Sources:

1. *Internet (do a search on Hepatitis)*
2. *Center for Disease and Control (CDC)*
3. *Massachusetts Department of Health*
4. *Beth Israel-Deaconess Hospital's Learning Center Boston, Massachusetts*
5. *Schering Corporation's patient educational video and pamplets on Intron.*
6. *American Liver Foundation, New England Chapter*
7. *Hepatitis Foundation International, Cedar Grove, NJ*

Questions and Answers About Hepatitis C

What is Hepatitis C?

In general, elevated liver enzymes and a positive antibody test for Hepatitis C Virus (HCV) means that an individual has Chronic Hepatitis C. However, the Anti-HCV may remain positive for several years after recovery from acute Hepatitis C, falsely indicating Chronic Hepatitis. In these two cases, liver enzymes are typically normal. The Hepatitis C virus was identified and described in 1989. In 1990, a Hepatitis C antibody test (Anti-HCV) became available commercially, to help identify individuals exposed to HCV. In 1992, a more specific test for Anti-HCV became available that better identified or confirmed the presence of the virus.

Chronic Hepatitis C appears to be a slowly progressive disease that gradually advances over ten to forty years. There is some evidence that the disease may progress faster when acquired in middle-age or later. In one study, Chronic Hepatitis found by liver biopsy was identified on the average of ten years following blood transfusions, and cirrhosis was found on an average of twenty years. It also appears that HCV, like the Hepatitis B virus, is associated with an increased chance of developing Hepatocellular Carcinoma, a type of primary liver cancer.

Almost all HCV-related liver cancer occurs with cirrhosis (scarring) of the liver. The exact magnitude of this risk is unknown but appears to be a late risk factor occurring on the average of thirty years after the time of infection. This is more prevalent in the Far East than in the United States.

Does Hepatitis C affect fertility?

No it does not. Women who are infected can still get pregnant and infected men can still impregnate women.

Can I Give the Disease to Others?

HCV can be transmitted through blood transfusions. However, all blood is now tested for the presence of this virus by the antibody test. It is estimated that the risk of post-transfusion Hepatitis C has been reduced by eight percent to ten percent. I.V. drug users, health care workers or laboratory technicians who may come in contact with infected blood, instruments, or needles are at a greater risk of acquiring Hepatitis C. Currently, there is no vaccine available to immunize individuals against this virus.

The risk for transmitting Hepatitis C sexually is unknown. There have been rare, documented cases of people with Chronic Hepatitis C transmitting the virus to their long-term sexual partner. The Center For Disease Control and Prevention (CDC) states that because of the lack of sufficient information, those with only one, long-term sexual partner need not change their sexual practices. Many physicians who counsel patients with Hepatitis C recommend the same thing.

The CDC says there is an increased risk of becoming infected with Hepatitis C if you have multiple sex partners. It is uncertain whether the use of latex condoms is 100% effective in preventing someone from infecting one's sexual partner or becoming infected themselves.

Is There a Treatment for Chronic Hepatitis C?

Interferon Alfa-2b is effective in the treatment of adults with Chronic Hepatitis C. The recommended dose of Interferon Alfa-2b for the treatment of Chronic Hepatitis C is 3,000,000 units, three times a week, administered by subcutaneous or intramuscular injection. Frequent blood tests are needed to monitor white blood cells, platelets and liver enzymes. A liver biopsy is typically done prior to treatment to determine the severity of liver damage and provide confirmation of the underlying disease. During the treatment period, the patient is monitored carefully for side effects including flu-like symptoms, depression, rashes, abnormal blood counts and other unusual reactions.

In a recent multi-center trial in Europe, forty-four percent of the Hepatitis C patients on the standard dosage for eighteen months had their elevated liver enzymes return to normal. This group was evaluated nineteen to forty-two months after this initial eighteen month treatment and half of them still had normal liver enzymes. The hope is that improvement or normalization of liver tests and reduced inflammation in the liver will slow or interrupt the development of progressive liver disease.

The results of several published clinical studies demonstrate that about fifty percent to seventy percent of patients with Chronic Hepatitis C respond to treatment with Interferon Alfa-2b. Several studies have also shown that about seventy percent of patients have a decrease in liver inflammation on follow-up liver biopsies.

Only ten to fifteen percent of patients treated with Interferon have a long-lasting response. Unfortunately, most patients relapse and have increases in liver inflammation after treatment is discontinued. Longer treatment periods and/or higher doses of Interferon Alfa-2b for patients with Chronic Hepatitis C who relapse, or do not respond to the recommended dose, are presently being evaluated in several approved clinical studies.

Patients can be treated a second time and eighty-five percent of patients will enter a second remission.

What Should I Do If I Test Positive for the Hepatitis C Virus?

Seek referral to a gastroenterologist or liver specialist. Further testing can be performed to determine the significance of the reactive antibody and whether or not one has Chronic Hepatitis C.

Chapter Three

Go all the way to the edge,
don't settle for a safe position.

Doctor Najarian - Finding a Cure for Chronic Hepatitis B

This chapter is intended to give insight into the life of Dr. Najarian. It is also intended to help one understand his reasoning and how he arrived at the decision to use the combination treatment of Interferon Alfa-2b and Ribavirin.

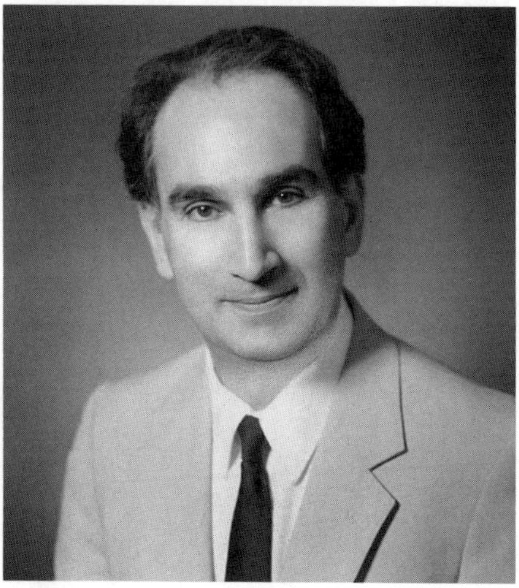

Dr. Thomas Najarian

EDUCATIONAL BACKGROUND
Dr. Najarian's partial educational background.

Dr. Najarian graduated from Harvard Medical School in 1974 with an M.D. degree. He was an intern and Resident in Medicine at the Boston Veteran's Administration (VA) Hospital in Boston, Massachusetts from 1974 to 1976. He was then chosen at Boston City Hospital to be part of the medical emergency team that was to take care of President Gerald Ford in case of an emergency while he was in Boston. Dr. Najarian was a fellow in Hematology at Boston V.A. Hospital, Boston, Massachusetts from 1977 to 1978, and also a board-certified specialist in Internal Medicine in 1978. He was included in Marquis Who's Who in the East 1981; and was inducted into the Academic Hall of Fame, Rockland High School, Massachusetts in 1990.

Dr. Najarian enrolled in the Massachusetts Institute of Technology in 1965 and graduated in 1970 with a S.B./S.M. combined degree in Mechanical Engineering.service award at graduation by the faculty for work in arranging a lecture series on environmental health.

PROFESSIONAL EXPERIENCE

Dr. Najarian has worked extensively with cancer and leukemia patients. Dr. Najarian has contributed greatly to the legalization of the combination treatment in Europe and United States. He was a staff physician at the Veterans Administration from 1979 to 1983, and Instructor in medicine at Boston University School of Medicine from 1979 to 1983. He has been a member of the staff of Mt. Auburn Hospital, Cambridge, Massachusetts since 1983 and has had a private practice of Internal Medicine since that time.

He is now specializing in the cure of Hepatitis C because he is confident that he can cure Hepatitis B.

More details of Dr. Najarian's professional experience and publications are given in the Appendix.

INTERVIEW WITH DR. NAJARIAN CONDUCTED BY KUNMI OLULEYE ON MONDAY APRIL 1, 1996.

This interview was conducted to give the reader a complete picture of Dr. Najarian. It was an opportunity to hear his feelings before, during and after the treatment. Even though some of the questions asked during the interview, do not relate directly to the cure of Hepatitis, they show the kind of person who would pursue and succeed prescribing an unconventional treatment.

Question: What interested you in becoming a doctor?
Answer: I have always been interested in science, astronomy, and engineering. I earned a degree in all except astronomy. There are many stories that led to my becoming a doctor, most of which are tragic. I am the kind

of person that if I put my mind to it, I can do just about anything. I have the ability to find obscure things.

STORY #1:

When I was a senior in high school, my sister became ill with Hodgkin's disease, which is a form of cancer of the lymph system. At the time, no one knew what caused it. It is still vague today what causes it. The treatment she received at M.G.H. (Massachusetts General Hospital) was partially effective. She suffered a relapse at the end of the treatment, but doctors led us to believe that she will be cured. I decided to help my family and sister deal with this disease and became involved in research at M.G.H. That's how I got into medicine.

STORY #2:

I took a course with Dr. Harriet Hardy in the field of Epidemiology - the study of what causes diseases, study of population. This was an extremely influential course in convincing me to pursue medicine.

STORY #3:

Sina *[Dr. Najarian's wife]*'s brother became deathly ill when I was in medical school. His white blood cell count was low, it went from 200-0, but he did not have AIDS. Remember how Ibi's was about 800? *[Kunmi: Yes.]* Well, Sina's brother was diagnosed with the disease of the polys (type of blood disease) and became sicker and sicker with infections. The doctors suggested he be treated with chemotherapy which I thought would have killed him. His Hematologist prescribed chemotherapy and a bone marrow transplant.

After much research reading through 25 years of monthly giant volumes of Index Medicus by hand, since there was no computer system at the time, I discovered that his profile fits that of Cyclic-Neutropenia, not Pre-Leukemic Syndrome. His white blood count was low one week of the month and stabilized for two weeks.

I found a paper written by a doctor in 1949 and Sina's brother fit the bill for one-third of his patients, in terms of age, genetic background, count cycle and so on. He was quite healthy when the poly count was 300, but within two weeks it would drop to zero. It is said that if one survives the disease for two years, one would be cured. At the time, there were experimental treatments with Androgens and Steroids to stabilize the condition and I suggested we try the treatment. He gradually stabilized within six months to one year, and has been fine ever since.

Question: Why did you feel the need to videotape Ibi's consultation session?
Answer: Paranoia and attention to detail. Two of my patients after I saw Ibi told me that with previous doctors, undergoing treatment, no warnings were given to them. I videotaped the session, to communicate the seriousness of the treatment, to emphasize to you how important it is to listen to these things. To make sure that the patient understands that this is a non-standard treatment.

Question: How did you feel when you started Ibi's treatment?
Answer: Very concerned. At my age, forty-eight, and in my career, I have not caused the death of a patient yet and it may happen someday. I wouldn't know how to deal with it. My attention to detail and persistence in monitoring my patient's health on a daily basis may be the reason why I haven't lost anyone yet. Some patients that were treated with the same or similar medications by other doctor's had bi-weekly or monthly visits. I couldn't do that in good conscience. This was a risky treatment.

Question: How do you feel now that the treatment is over?
Answer: Relief!! We could have lost him, or done severe permanent medical damage—we came close. Ibi got the highest dose of the treatment. The most nerve-wracking time was after the treatment was over and the blood count came back really low. I had asked Ibi to come in immediately for another test which I personally spun and it looked normal, before I sent it off to the lab. My personality is really compulsive about all my patient's results. Am I killing the bone marrow, etc.. I was extremely panicky at the time and I caused my whole family to have anxiety attacks.

Question: Is there a bond with Ibi or any other patients?
Answer: [Laughed, then smiled and he repeated the question.] Of course, I have a bond with all my patients. I want to cure every one of them. I am very protective of their care and them personally. I get disappointed when my patients leave me for health insurance coverage reasons. I guess they don't share the same sentiment for me as I do for them. I can understand their financial need to go with the cheapest insurance plan. Most of the time, the insurance plan does not provide adequate coverage for them. Some companies limit the care doctors give their patient - there's a limit to the number of MRIs, X-rays or tests the patient can have in a calendar year.

I cannot belong to any one of those and therefore lose that patient. Most doctors nowadays work for hospitals because they cannot keep up with all the new rules and regulations various insurance plans declare every so often, besides there are so many of them. It's hard to keep track of the paperwork.

The treatment for Ibi is over, but there are others underway for which I am cautiously optimistic. I intend to make this my life's work.

Question: What are you focusing on now?
Answer: The cure for liver cancer of which Hepatitis B and C are causes. Also the confirmation of my discovered cure for Hepatitis C. I am trying to get more Hepatitis C patients to treat. After I have cured ten patients, then I can go public with the information. Even though B is more prevalent and I am convinced that I can cure it, C is more challenging.

Some doctors are developing more confidence in me and I am getting referrals from them. The Phlebotomy, which is taking blood out of the system to reduce the iron level in the body is now becoming a standard part of this combination treatment in hospitals, such as Massachusetts General Hospital, one of the hospitals Schering Corporation is using for their studies.

Question: What were the key elements in making this treatment successful?
Answer: An informed and intelligent patient, vitamins, and a dedicated doctor with concrete and carefully monitored plans.

Please refer to the Appendix for the remaining interview with Dr. Najarian.

DR. NAJARIAN'S MEDICAL NOTES AND DOCUMENTATION OF THE COMBINATION TREATMENT.

Several studies (see #1 and #2 under reference on p. 37) have shown synergistic effects in curing Hepatitis C with a combination of Interferon-Alfa and Ribavirin. Ribavirin has been shown to inhibit the Hepatitis B virus (see #3), and in combination with Interferon-Beta (see #4) to cure two out of eight patients. Interferon-Alfa in the dosage range of ten million units TIW (three times a week) will result in virologic cure in about forty percent of cases. I report a virology cure of Chronic Hepatitis B with a combination of Interferon-Alfa and Ribavirin.

A 100 kilogram (218 pounds) Nigerian male in his early thirties, Ibiyinka Oluleye was presented to me with at least a four-year history of elevated liver enzymes and positive results for Hepatitis B surface antigen and B e-antigen. When therapy with Interferon-Alfa was explained to him he wished to have an improved chance of cure if possible and agreed to treatment. His initial white blood count was 3,800/mcL with 1500 neutrophilis. Initial ferritin level was 614 ng/ML. Liver enzymes were fifty to 100 percent above normal, but liver function was normal.

At the start of treatment with Interferon-alfa, ten million units SC TIW (this means under the skin, three times a week) and Ribavirin 600 mg po bid, the patient was also phlebotomized one unit of blood weekly for six weeks. Phlebotomy was stopped after an MRI of the liver was normal with no increase in iron stores. The patient also took MVI one daily, Vitamin C 1,000 mg/day and Vitamin E 400 U/day. Despite the phlebotomy and Ribavirin, his hematocrit value never went below thirty-six, and in fact returned to the low forties throughout treatment after phlebotomy was stopped.

Five weeks into treatment, his WBC fell to 1,840, his newtrophils fell to 700/mcL, and platelets to 116,000 /cmm. G-CSF (booster hormone), 300 mcg SC TIW was then started and given about six hours before each

Interferon injection. His WBC (white blood count) subsequently ranged between 3,000 and 23,000 with about sixty percent netrophils. His platelet count also rose to normal on treatment. His Hepatitis B e-antigen was negative at eight weeks, his liver enzymes flared two to three times normal at twelve weeks and subsequently declined to normal after treatment. His Hepatitis B surface antigen became negative at sixteen weeks of treatment, and at twenty weeks when his Hepatitis B DNA by PCR was negative, treatment was stopped.

Treatment was well tolerated, with most of the side effects of flu-like symptoms caused by Interferon. Interestingly, when the WBC was very low, the side effects from Interferon almost disappeared, only to return after the G-CSF was administered, suggesting that perhaps a normal number of white blood count is needed for Interferon to work.

References:

1. Brillanti S., Garson J., Foli M., et al. *A Pilot Study of Combination Therapy With Ribavirin Plus Interferon Alfa-2b for Interferon Alfa-resistant Chronic Hepatitis C.* Gastroenterology Vol. 107 (3): pp. 812-7, September 1994.
2. Lai M.Y., Yang P.M., Kao J.T., et al. *Combination Therapy of a-Interferon and Ribavirin In Patients With Chronic Hepatitis C: An Interim Report.* AASLD abstracts, Hepatology 1993 Oct; 18(4) Pt 2: p.146.
3. Fried M.W., Fong G.L., Swain M.G., et al. "Therapy of Chronic Hepatitis B with a Six-month Course of Ribavirin." J. Hepatology 1994 Aug; 21(2): pp. 145-50.
4. Kakumu S., Yoshioka K., Wakita T., et al. "Pilot study of Ribavirin and Interferon-Beta for Chronic Hepatitis B." Hepatology 1993 Aug; 18(2): pp. 258-63.

Chapter Four

Freedom comes with understanding who you are.

Treatment, Nutrition, Coping and Caring

The following pages will take you into a five-month (January to May 1995) daily journal of our lives. Ibi's daily intake: food, drugs (Ribavirin & Interferon Alfa-2b), vitamins, and later toward the middle of the treatment, the booster hormone (G-CSF) was added. Ribavirin and Vitamins were taken orally, while the Interferon and hormone were injected.

You will read about how I, Kunmi, cared for him and coped during those months.

Since this is *not* a medical textbook, only *certain lab results are listed in the Appendix* to avoid distraction from the main theme, which is our experience with Chronic Hepatitis B.

The journal raises many interesting questions, for example nutrition. Was Ibi on a special diet? No, he was not. He could eat anything and as much of it as he wanted. Does nutrition have an impact on the treatment? In this case, it is hard to determine. Many of his food intakes were high carbohydrate, low protein meals, especially the Nigerian Cuisines. All the Quaker Oats entries refer to Oatmeal. The tables will sometimes have multiple entries of the same dish or unusual breakfast entries, this is not a misprint, it is what he ate. No exercise or physical therapy was prescribed with the treatment.

At the time of the treatment Ibi worked as an Environmental Health and Safety Specialist at a university in Boston. To give you an idea of his daily schedule, his work hours were usually from eight a.m. to five-thirty p.m. His job was to make sure the university was in compliance with state and federal radiation safety regulations. This involved a lot of walking, visiting labs, technicians and faculty. It also involved responding to chemical spills and other accidents in the labs.

There was so much information that Ibi was unable to record in his journal due to his medication. For example, he had two turtles as pets and changes their water every two to three days; only one entry reflects this. He also left out other entries because he forgot about them. So as you read, if you come across entries that seem incomplete, it is due to this reason.

Many of the journal entries were written as they occur, others were finished the next day. For example, on page 85 when Ibi talked about planning for the future, he wrote many of his thoughts down that night, he then fell asleep and completed the entry in the morning. Excerpt from page 85, February 23's entry: *"I would like many great things in my future......I fell asleep."*

The first week of treatment was the worst. I made brief entries and Ibi made none.

Wednesday, January 18 - Saturday, January 21

Kunmi's Entry

Ibi was in no condition to make entries and I was in a state of panic and anxiety. He had severe headaches, pains, and fever. He could not sleep and therefore kept me up most of the night. He sees things that are not there. We had to call Dr. Najarian during the night, around three or four a.m. when things became unbearable. He told Ibi to take some Tylenol, and an hour later Ibi was sleeping soundly. Ibi took Tylenol at night for the entire week. This happened for all four days.

Sunday, January 22

Kunmi's Entry

It was a dreadful, rainy day. Ibi was cranky and complained about every single thing. He complained about my driving, so I pulled over and asked if he wanted to drive. He said nothing and I continued driving. He was less cranky later in the evening.

Monday, January 23

Kunmi's Entry

Ibi said he felt fine in the morning although he looked extremely tired. He is not talking much, but has a good appetite, and eats a lot. This is the best that he has been since the treatment began on January 18. I am too busy watching him to write a more detailed journal entry.

TUESDAY, JANUARY 24

Kunmi's Entry

Ibi was dehydrated and drank lots of water in the middle of the night. He did not have much of an appetite and complained all night of aches or pains, groaning constantly.

WEDNESDAY, JANUARY 25

Ibi's Entry

I woke up feeling normal with no sign of medicinal side effects. I had lunch around 1:30 p.m. I visited my doctor at 5:30 p.m. for my weekly checkup. He informed me of that the liver enzyme level needs to increase at the beginning of the treatment, then decrease.

He took a pint of blood because the level of iron was high in my system. Blood contains iron. The high iron level would prevent the medication from working. Removing the blood reduces the iron level because there is that much less blood in the body.

	Breakfast	Lunch	Dinner
	Large bowl of Quaker Oats, cranberry juice	Chicken breast broccoli, carrots, yogurt, chicken pot pie, and an apple	Rice and fish stew
Medications	600 mg of Ribavirin		.2cc Interferon 600 mg of Ribavirin
Vitamins	500 mg of C, 400IU of E, Multi-Vitamin		500 mg of C

Kunmi's Entry

I went with Ibi for his weekly checkup. The needle was quite big, but Ibi was brave. I held his hand, and distracted him from noticing as the needle pierced his arm. I felt the pain, even though it was not my arm it went into.

On the way home, we bought his multi-vitamins, one without Iron, Vitamin C and E. He took another dose of Interferon. Ibi put dishes in the dishwasher.

THURSDAY, JANUARY 26

Ibi's Entry

I woke up this morning with a sharp pain on the left side of my chest. If I lean to the right it hurts, and it also hurts if I breathe in at a particular posture. The pain was still there at the end of the day, but it was bearable. I called my doctor and told him about the pain, because he said not to hide anything from him.

Dr. Najarian told me to go to Sancta Maria Hospital in Cambridge to have a chest x-ray taken, which I did. He later told me that my last blood test revealed that my white blood cell count was low. He said I should reduce the Interferon to .1cc three times a week until my white count is higher. He made an appointment for me to see him on Friday at 7:45 a.m. to draw blood for another white blood count.

	Breakfast	Lunch	Dinner
	Quaker Oats	An apple and yogurt	Corned beef stew with bread
Medications	600 mg of Ribavirin		600 mg of Ribavirin
Vitamins	500 mg of C, 400IU of E, Multi-Vitamin		500 mg of C

Kunmi's Entry

Ibi picked Sayo up from school after his chest x-ray.

FRIDAY, JANUARY 27

Ibi's Entry

I woke up in the morning with pain on the left side of my chest. I left home at 7:30 a.m. for my appointment with Doctor Najarian. I had breakfast and took my medications. Dr. Najarian took blood to check the white cell count. I had a small sandwich for lunch which I did not feel like eating but my stomach felt empty. My work went on normally for the rest of the day, and I felt normal except for the pain in the left side of my chest. I called my doctor at about four p.m. for the results of my blood test. The count was the same as the last time, and my hemoglobin was a little lower than before, which was expected.

Kunmi's son, Sayo and I went to the mall for dinner after I picked him up at school. I bought two chicken meals for my fiancée for her dinner. I ate all of my food and Sayo's leftovers. When we came home, Sayo went to watch TV and I went to my room to inject my medication.

It feels easier to inject myself now. In the beginning I was uncomfortable with the idea of inserting a needle into my body, by myself. I prefer the medication be injected by an experienced medical person. I did not feel sick from the Interferon injection.

I went to sleep very early because I was tired. When my fiancée came back home, she sat on the bed and ate her dinner. I became hungry watching her eat and she spoon-fed me as she ate. It felt good to be a kid again. After that I stayed up for a while before I fell asleep.

	Breakfast	Lunch	Dinner
	Quaker Oats	Tuna sandwich	Vegetarian delight from Japanese fast food
Medications	600 mg of Ribavirin		.1cc Interferon, 600 mg of Ribavirin
Vitamins	500 mg of C, 400IU of E, Multi-Vitamin		500 mg of C

Kunmi's Entry

Ibi went to see Dr. Najarian. The Interferon dose was decreased to .1cc and the x-rays were fine. His appetite certainly has returned, but he looked tired and said he was tired. He was asleep in bed with the TV on when I arrived. As I sat down with my dinner to watch him sleep, he woke up. I borrowed a herbal nutrition book which lists appropriate herbs and vegetable for various diseases, including hepatitis. I hope to find out how I can better help Ibi in terms of cooking the right foods, and learning how the vitamins he is taking help his treatment.

SATURDAY, JANUARY 28

Ibi's Entry

After Kunmi left for school, I cleaned up the kitchen and the living room. The house we bought is almost seventy years old and needs a lot of work. The gas company contractors came to repair the boiler, which has stopped working. The windows are extremely drafty which results in high heating and cooling cost. I oversaw the work of the contractors from the replacement window and gas company.

After the contractors left, I read the manual for the installation of Lotus Notes, then went out with my wife to do some shopping. When we came back home, I took my medication and then we went to sleep.

	Breakfast	Lunch	Dinner
	Chicken and Rice	Chicken and Rice	Chicken, onion rings, grape juice and lots of water
Medications	600 mg of Ribavirin		600 mg of Ribavirin
Vitamins	500 mg of C, 400IU of E, Multi-Vitamin		500 mg of C

Kunmi's Entry

I had to go to finance class review at 8:30 a.m., so I couldn't fix breakfast for the boys. I'm sure they'll take care of themselves. I came home at four p.m., and the kitchen was spotless — the boys were fed. This assured me that Ibi was fine.

Later we went to an African restaurant to discuss a possible rental for our September 3 wedding. We liked the place. Ibi was his quiet self, and I did most of the talking. He looked a bit tired and somewhat irritated. We later went to a supermarket. We came home, and I cooked chicken for Ibi me, pizza for Sayo and fish for tomorrow's dinner. Ibi ate dinner and drank lots of water.

We later watched a movie. Ibi developed a fever about nine p.m. He fell asleep and when I touched him after ten p.m., the fever was gone. He did not take any medication so I wondered what reduced the fever.

SUNDAY, JANUARY 29

Ibi's Entry

It felt like the beginning of a good day. I did some handyman's work around the house such as filling cracks in the wall with foam sealants. I was so occupied that I took my medication and vitamins late. Then I ate breakfast and read the Sunday newspapers. I went to the hardware store to buy more sealant for filling holes and cracks in the walls. I continued the work when I got back home. I was quite happy for being physically able to do so much work. In the evening, we went to Kunmi's friend's house for a homemade Chinese dinner. The food was delicious, so I ate a lot. I took my medication around 8:30 p.m. and went straight to bed.

	Breakfast	Lunch	Dinner
	Bread and eggs two cups of hot chocolate	Clam chowder and crackers	Chinese food
Medications	600 mg of Ribavirin		600 mg of Ribavirin
Vitamins	500 mg of C, 400IU of E, Multi-Vitamin		500 mg of C

Kunmi's Entry

We woke up early, six a.m. Ibi and I read the paper looking for a new gas stove for our tenant. They live upstairs in our other three-bedroom unit. A family with their two children, a boy and a girl. Prior to Ibi's treatment, I had mentioned to the couple that Ibi has Hepatitis B, and asked if it was okay for Sayo to stay with them sometimes in the evening until I get home. They were familiar with Hepatitis because their daughter had Hepatitis A and was cured. She got it from drinking the water during a vacation in Bolivia. They were supportive and were willing to keep Sayo to help relieve Ibi. I was glad that they were educated about the disease and had no fear of it.

We filled some of the cracks and I put the pink insulation stuff in the roof. Ibi filled most of the cracks in the walls and windows. He wasn't tired and we finished at 2:30 p.m.

We went to my friend and business school classmate, CC, for Chinese New Year. I didn't have the right apartment so Ibi was upset with me. He was more upset than usual and I wondered if it had anything to do with the medication. I apologized and said very little to not annoy him any further. We finally found it while visiting Alima, my Cameroonian friend who lives in the same building and, coincidentally, on the same floor.

We came home at seven p.m. and Ibi was exhausted.

MONDAY, JANUARY 30

Ibi's Entry

I woke up okay. I ironed my clothes, got in the shower, dressed, and took my medication with some cranberry juice. Then I left home for work and had lunch around 1:30 p.m. I was feeling bored and needed a distraction. Whenever I get bored I really feel the effect of the medication. I decided to go to my old workplace at Harvard and pick up the books I left there. It was good to see old co-workers and friends. They were glad to see me too. When I got back to the office, I did some work for the budget. I had a nice day at work; it was not stressful things went at a slow pace.

Later I went to pick Sayo up at school. We both had dinner, and I took my medication. I tried to resolve the backup tape configuration problem on the home computer. It took a long while to figure out the problem. I backed up some files on the backup tape. I went to bed around eleven p.m. after taking my injection. I felt a little feverish and achy, but it was very mild.

	Breakfast	Lunch	Dinner
	Cranberry juice	Whopper meal - burger, fries and soda	Rice and turkey stew
Medications	600 mg of Ribavirin		.2cc Interferon 600 mg of Ribavirin
Vitamins	500 mg of C, 400IU of E, Multi-Vitamin		500 mg of C

Kunmi's Entry

My brother M.T. and Ibi talked about him working on M.T.'s network. Ibi was quite excited about the opportunity. I was excited too. This will not only keep him occupied, he will also be gaining a skill that will make him very marketable.

Ibi seemed okay today. He had no temper tantrums or irritations. I had to stay in school late, so Ibi picked Sayo up from school. He fed him and put him to bed.

When I got home, I found Ibi working on the

computer, backing up software to a tape drive. He was trying to backup files on the computer prior to reformatting it.

On my way home, I bought scratch tickets. Ibi helped me scratch them after finishing his work on the computer. We won twenty-five dollars.

TUESDAY, JANUARY 31

Ibi's Entry

I was in good condition after last night's rest. I didn't feel feverish, and there were no aches and pains. I took my medication and left for work. It was a busy day at work since I had to meet with my director to justify my computer network proposal's high quote. I was asked to write an estimate for the computer networking system that I suggest, which we desperately need. I spent a lot of time on the phone with vendors trying to get quotes. I picked the most cost-effective component from the vendor who gave the best price and ended up with more than one vendor for the entire network system. This is similar to building a house from scratch, with the owner acting as the general contractor, subcontracting to other handymen depending on their speciality.

My director was really annoying me. We need this system in place and he wants to be penny wise, pound foolish. I later talked to my immediate manager about what can be done to cut down the cost. Since I have been allocated funds for a notebook computer, I decided to apply that money to the cost of the network. I left work around 6:15 p.m., had dinner, took my medication and went to bed around eight p.m.

	Breakfast	Lunch	Dinner
	Hot chocolate and one hot dog bun	Thai food	Chicken and yellow squash
Medications	600 mg of Ribavirin		600 mg of Ribavirin
Vitamins	500 mg of C, 400IU of E, Multi-Vitamin		500 mg of C

Kunmi's Entry

I stayed home today. Ibi called me from work to tell me about his lunch with his manager at a Thai restaurant. He was upset about his discussion with his manager and the director about his network proposal.

Ibi and I ate dinner and talked more about how the day went. He was still upset and I reminded him that he needs to try to not let things get to him because of his medication. Ibi went to bed exhausted at eight p.m. I was up until after ten p.m. partly to watch him sleep and see if he develops a fever or any other reactions. He seemed to have had a hard day. Ibi must not have been sleeping soundly because he woke up a few times as I moved around the room.

I sat on the bed, felt his temperature and it seemed normal, no fever. I read a little, continued to watch Ibi, but fell asleep myself.

Chapter Five

Knowing the problem
is half the solution.

Wednesday, February 1

Ibi's Entry

I woke up in good condition. I ironed my clothes, had my breakfast and took my medication before I left for work. I had a safety seminar in Downtown Boston, but I couldn't drive in, so I took the train. It felt strange because it's been such a long time since I have taken the train. The seminar was boring and disorganized. I went back to the office after the seminar for the rest of the day.

I went for my appointment with Dr. Najarian at 5:45 p.m. My wife met me at the doctor's office. He took some blood for testing and measured my blood pressure. It was okay, so he drew one pint of blood to reduce my iron level. He gave me some grapefruit juice to quench my thirst.

His wife gave us some homemade soup. She made it out of chicken broth and sweet yams. It tasted really good and it was my first time trying this kind of soup. She gave us one gallon of it to take home. Later I took my second round of medications and vitamins.

	Breakfast	Lunch	Dinner
	Quaker Oats	Tuna sandwich, grapefruit juice and a chocolate bar	Grapefruit juice, chicken broth and sweet yam soup, Whopper meal - burger, fries and soda
Medications	600 mg of Ribavirin		600 mg of Ribavirin
Vitamins	500 mg of C, 400IU of E, Multi-Vitamin		500 mg of C

Kunmi's Entry

After Ibi got dressed this morning, he asked for my approval, and I said he looked very handsome. This was unusual because he rarely asked how he looks. Prior to now, he gets dressed, looks in the mirror and tells himself how gorgeous he is and how lucky I am to have him. I teased him by asking if he really was off to a seminar or business meeting, and he laughed. It was such a pleasure to see that old familiar smile.

I stayed home again today because I felt that it was time for me to rest. The last few weeks have been quite an ordeal emotionally and physically.

Ibi went to see Dr. Najarian, who drew one pint of blood. It was quicker this time because the blood pressure machine was wrapped around Ibi's arm and pumped before the needle was inserted. I held the blood pressure pump so that the pressure stayed at a particular level. Ibi's blood pressure was normal, but it was high last week. I asked Dr. Najarian about what happens to the blood he takes from Ibi every week and he said that it is disposed by the lab company that he deals with. Since the blood is contaminated, it can't be used for anything.

Ibi ate only one whopper for dinner. I expected him to eat two, which he normally does in minutes. He felt good with his conversation with M.T. in getting involved with M.T.'s company. He wasn't cranky, he was actually quite jovial. I wondered if it was because I felt rested and ready to tackle what may come, or if he was as happy as he seemed.

THURSDAY, FEBRUARY 2

Ibi's Entry

I woke up in good health. Dr. Najarian told me to call him at ten a.m. for the results of my blood test, but I could not call him until about two p.m. because I was so busy at work. When I talked to him, he said my white blood cell count was low when the treatment started, and still is. He told me to return to the 0.2cc dose for the Interferon injection. He said I should not use it on Wednesday, before my next meeting with him. He said I should use it on Thursday, to change the days that I administer my doses. I took my Ribavirin and vitamin for the evening, and had dinner. I could not fall asleep for a long time. Kunmi helped occupy the time with her school issues. We later play-wrestled and I was able to fall asleep.

	Breakfast	Lunch	Dinner
	Quaker Oats	Skipped lunch	One whopper and spaghetti
Medications	600 mg of Ribavirin		600 mg of Ribavirin
Vitamins	500 mg of C, 400IU of E, Multi-Vitamin		500 mg of C

Kunmi's Entry

I warmed yesterday's leftover Quaker Oats for Ibi's breakfast. I was eager to hear the results of the blood tests. I was a bit worried at one p.m. when I had not heard from Ibi, so I called him. I was even more concerned to learn the result, because the low count was not good.

Got home at ten p.m. He showed no sign of sleep. I assumed that he might be worried about the blood result. I didn't ask him because if he was not thinking about it and if there was something to worry about, there would be no point reminding him of it.

At 11:30 p.m., I decided that it was time for both of us to sleep. I switched the TV off, he turned the light off. He wanted the TV back on and I wanted the light on, but dimmed. I turned the light back on and he turned the TV back on, so we play-wrestled — this went on for 20 minutes, eventually he moved the lamp out of the room as I went to hide the TV's remote control. I later searched for the lamp and I couldn't find it, so I turned the light in the next room on. He searched for the remote control. He got tired and we both went to bed. This was fun and he was able to sleep.

FRIDAY, FEBRUARY 3

Ibi's Entry

I awoke and in good health, took my morning round of medication. What a boring day it was at work. I did a lot of moving around on campuses. Part of my job is to make sure that the labs are in compliance with state and federal safety regulations, so I occassionally visit the labs for this reason.

The department had a retirement party for a colleague. There was a lot to eat and I ate at least three plates of various things.

I got home around 6:30 p.m. I watched a movie and read information on a computer platform called UNIX. This is the new field that I am considering pursuing, the opportunity offered to me in M.T.'s company. I later took my medication for the second part of the day.

	Breakfast	Lunch	Dinner
	Rice and stew	Cold cuts, hors d'oeuvres, chocolate cake	Nigerian Cuisine - Amala and Apon stew with stockfish
Medications	600 mg of Ribavirin		.2cc Interferon 600 mg of Ribavirin
Vitamins	500 mg of C, 400IU of E, Multi-Vitamin		500 mg of C

Kunmi's Entry

He was in high spirits today. I found the lamp in the kitchen by the stove the next morning, neatly tucked into a corner. Ibi was quite pleased with himself because he successfully hid something from me. He smiled all morning every time he looked at me. I let him enjoy the moment.

I came home at 9:30 p.m. and he was in bed. He had a slight temperature around eleven p.m. He told me about the party at work and all that he did and ate, hot and cold hors d'oeuvres, chocolate cake, the apple cider from heaven, etc. He resumed an injection of 0.2cc of Interferon.

SATURDAY, FEBRUARY 4

Ibi's Entry

Woke up okay, cleaned the house. Took my medication. Ten inches of snow had fallen since yesterday evening. Kunmi went to school in the morning. We went shopping before the start of the next snowstorm which was to happen that night.

Kunmi dragged me with her to the wedding dressmaker to adjust her wedding dress. I went to my barber for a haircut. He thought I was crazy coming in for a haircut in the snowstorm. When we came back home we had been plowed out of the house. We had to dig our way into the driveway. It took an hour to shovel out enough snow to create a pathway. I was exhausted and cold. I went in and took my medication for the day. We had dinner and I felt a fever coming on, so I went to sleep.

	Breakfast	Lunch	Dinner
	Quaker Oats	Turkey sandwich with bacon, lettuce and tomato	Chicken, rice, vegetables and gravy
Medications	600 mg of Ribavirin		600 mg of Ribavirin
Vitamins	500 mg of C, 400IU of E, Multi-Vitamin		500 mg of C

Kunmi's Entry

Ibi looked tired today. Even though the weather was horrible, I felt that he needed to go out. So we took my wedding dress to my friend's mother who is a dressmaker in Jamaica Plain, Massachusetts. I regretted stepping out of the house on that dreadful snowy Saturday from the minute we left.

After leaving the dressmaker, Ibi went to the barber at two p.m. and dropped Sayo and me off at my sister's in Lynn. Ibi came back from the barber at three p.m. very cold, saying that he was developing a fever. He asked for and drank a big mug of hot tea.

We came home to find two feet of snow blocking the driveway. The city's snow plow had plowed us in with the snow they cleared off the street. I felt that they could have put the snow somewhere else. We shoveled. I did most of the work. Ibi is to be commended because he really tried in shoveling the little that he did considering his condition.

Ibi put the ice melt in the driveway and the pathway. He started having chest pains once the shoveling was over. He had to lie down on the bed once we got in. He then started saying "I know you don't care" over and over. So I went and lay next to him, pulling him closer, like a mother does her child. I stroked his forehead and he fell asleep.

Later that evening, when Ibi woke up, he continued to complain of chest pains and needed to stay in bed. I brought his dinner into the bedroom and he couldn't feed himself. He kept dropping the spoon, so I had to feed him. He started feeling nauseated at eight p.m., but he didn't have a temperature. He stayed in bed exhausted. After pampering him a bit, I nagged him for shoveling snow when he knew his condition. I told him I would have understood if he had stopped shoveling earlier than he did. He developed a high fever at 9:30 p.m.

The fever got worse and one of the wonderful moments of this treatment occurred. I went into the kitchen to make Ibi a cup of tea to take with Tylenol and Sayo was watching TV in the living room. He asked if Daddy was okay because he noticed that Ibi had been in the bedroom for a while and quiet. I told Sayo that Daddy had a fever. He stopped watching TV and went into the bedroom. When I entered, Sayo was hugging Ibi in the cutest way. Both had their heads touching at the forehead, and Sayo was rubbing the back of Ibi's head, like I do to both of them. I just stood at the door and watched and smiled. My heart melted from such a display of love.

I gave Ibi his tea and Tylenol and got into bed. I fell asleep, but kept waking up throughout the night to check Ibi's condition. His fever was gone at three a.m.

SUNDAY, FEBRUARY 5

Ibi's Entry

I felt better this morning, but I thought I was going to die last night. I have no fever and mild chest pains. I managed to clean the house, read the Sunday papers and do some reading on the Internet.

It's been such a cold weekend, and I wanted to know if both cars worked today instead of waiting until tomorrow morning to find out. So in the evening I started the cars, but Kunmi's car would not start. We called our motor club for a jump start and after the jump, I saw there was little gas in the tank. I drove the car out to get gas and some starch for my clothes. When I got home I ironed my clothes for work.

	Breakfast	Lunch	Dinner
	Horlicks beverage, bread and fried eggs	Rice and turkey stew with vegetables	Rice and turkey stew with vegetables
Medications	600 mg of Ribavirin		600 mg of Ribavirin
Vitamins	500 mg of C, 400IU of E, Multi-Vitamin		500 mg of C

Kunmi's Entry

I slept late. It was ten a.m. when I woke up. Ibi had no fever in the morning. He looked very tired but was jovial. He volunteered to make breakfast after I started making it, but I did not let him.

I joined in with the house cleaning and was very tired after doing one load of laundry. I went back to sleep at one p.m. and woke up at 5:30 p.m.

I commend Ibi for going out in below zero degree weather to put gas in my car. When he got back, he looked very tired. He got himself ready for tomorrow's workday and went to bed. I felt his head as he slept and he had developed a fever. Since he was asleep, I didn't wake him to take Tylenol.

MONDAY, FEBRUARY 6

Ibi's Entry

I woke up, took a bath, as well as my medication, on an empty stomach and left for work. When we were about to leave home, Kunmi tried to start her car but it wouldn't start. We tried to jump start it but that didn't work either. She had to drop me at work so she could have the car. I think she took the day off at work to get it fixed. We decided that I could drop the car at the mechanic the next day.

Well, she changed all the plans and dropped me off at work. At around one p.m., I began to feel really hungry and went to a send-off party at work for one of my co-workers. I was still hungry after leaving because there was not much I felt like eating. So I went to the campus cafeteria and ate lunch there. It was good.

Kunmi picked me up at work at about 5:15 p.m. I came home, gave myself an injection, and took my second round of medication for the day. I listened to the news and read some information on Lotus Notes, a groupware application program.

	Breakfast	Lunch	Dinner
	Quaker Oats	Pork ribs with mashed potato, corn and green beans	Three hot dogs and three sweet bread rolls
Medications	600 mg of Ribavirin		.2cc Interferon 600 mg of Ribavirin
Vitamins	500 mg of C, 400IU of E, Multi-Vitamin		500 mg of C

Kunmi's Entry

Ibi looked very tired. I advised him to stay home and rest, but he refused.

Today was a waste. I stayed home and rested. Later, I picked Ibi and Sayo up from their respective places. I had no interest in cooking dinner, so I fed them hot dogs. We all went to bed at 7:30 p.m.

Ibi had a high temperature again.

TUESDAY, FEBRUARY 7

Ibi's Entry

I woke up and felt exhausted. I thought about taking the day off, but I found enough courage to go to work. I took a bath and medication on an empty stomach. The day was very busy, and I almost skipped lunch too. I had lunch at 12 p.m. and had to rush to a seminar in downtown Boston. The seminar was very informative.

I picked Sayo up at school and was told he was misbehaving. He was not listening in class. The teacher had to put him on time-out after speaking to him several times about his behavior. I explained to Sayo how in my culture, the teacher is one's parent for those hours that one is in school. Behaviors that are not acceptable at home, are also not acceptable at school. I explained our high expectations of him, which we believe he is capable of achieving because he is an intelligent boy. I asked why he behaved as he did and he gave no reason, but promised not to do it again. We came home and Sayo had two hot dogs. I had dinner also. I took my medication and lay down on my bed extremely tired.

	Breakfast	Lunch	Dinner
	Skipped breakfast	Spaghetti and meatballs	Hot chocolate and a large bowl of Quaker Oats
Medications	600 mg of Ribavirin		600 mg of Ribavirin
Vitamins	500 mg of C, 400IU of E, Multi-Vitamin		500 mg of C

Kunmi's Entry

Ibi complained about fatigue but he didn't want to call in sick because he was going to a seminar. I packed his lunch. I am very worried because he looks tired, enough to fall asleep at the wheel. I argued, saying all that I could think of to convince him to stay home, but he didn't.

I beeped Ibi several times today and got worried when he did not call me back. I called the office's main switchboard and was told that he was out somewhere on the campus. I hoped that he found a place to take a nap. He returned my call late in the afternoon and said that he was busy and tired and had decided to find somewhere to rest. I told him I was scared to death when he did not call right away, and he apologized. I suspect that he is depressed and did not want to talk about it. Severe depression is one of the side effects of Interferon.

Wednesday, February 8

Ibi's Entry

The day started good, but I was a little tired. I was starving though and had a big breakfast before going to work. I was very busy at work so I ate a chocolate crunch bar around one p.m. and had a late lunch. At about 5:10 p.m., I left work to see my doctor. He said he was glad that I was doing fine. He is the first doctor I ever had in the United States of America that had real and genuine concern for his patients' health. He also quite knowledgeable. He took my blood pressure, which he does at every visit. He checked my eyes and said they were okay. He also checked my vision and said I might want to have another test for my vision performed by another doctor later on.

Dr. Najarian suggested doing an AIDS test because my white blood count was still low. He told me he is positive that I don't have AIDS but would like to conduct a routine exam to confirm it. I was very concerned of the result. I hope it is negative. If it is positive, that's my confirmed death sentence. I don't think that I would want to continue the hepatitis treatment. I did not discuss this fear with Dr. Najarian. He asked me to sign a consent form for the AIDS test and I did.

He took one pint of blood as part of my weekly test, which was to reduce my iron and to help the drugs work better. He spun it in the centrifuge and my hemoglobin was okay. He mentioned that he missed my wife helping with this. Usually, she would play nurse while the doctor attended to my other issues. She usually holds the blood pressure machine as the blood pint bag fills up. She keeps me company, talking and joking, before you know it, the bag is full and it's time to go home. I miss her too on these visits.

After Dr. Najarian drew some blood, his wife prepared a plate of dinner for me. They invited me upstairs to eat the soup and I accepted their invitation. The doctor and I talked for some time while his wife worked in the kitchen. I left for home about 7:45 p.m. I felt really exhausted and went to sleep.

	Breakfast	Lunch	Dinner
	Two cups of hot chocolate, rice and stew	Rice with carrots and cauliflower, chocolate crunch bar	Wheat soup
Medications	600 mg of Ribavirin		600 mg of Ribavirin
Vitamins	500 mg of C, 400IU of E, Multi-Vitamin		500 mg of C

Kunmi's Entry

Very busy day from start to finish. Ibi walked in as I was about to call Dr. Najarian to find out if Ibi was with him. I asked why his appointment took so long. Was anything wrong? He said no. It took longer to draw the blood, since I was not there to help. He looked really down and exhausted. I wondered why, but left him alone.

THURSDAY, FEBRUARY 9

Ibi's Entry

I woke up well rested. I ate breakfast, then left for work. I had to interview a work-study student for a temporary position in my office, so I ate lunch around one p.m. Later, I called my doctor to find out the results of my blood test. He said it had not arrived yet. I did what I needed to do at work and picked Sayo up at school.

I called my doctor when I got home, and he told me that I should stay on the 0.2cc Interferon. He said he saw a slight improvement in my liver. That got my hopes a little bit higher. This was the best news I had all day.

I cleaned the kitchen and cut up the whole turkey in the refrigerator. I fed Sayo rice and ate some too. I took my injection, medicine, and vitamins, then watched TV to calm my nerves.

I will take Friday off to get some rest. I feel exhausted emotionally and physically.

	Breakfast	Lunch	Dinner
	Rice and stew strawberry yogurt, grapefruit and apple	Steak dinner with mixed vegetables and a roll	Rice, vegetables and stew
Medications	600 mg of Ribavirin		.2cc Interferon, 600 mg of Ribavirin
Vitamins	500 mg of C, 400IU of E, Multi-Vitamin		500 mg of C

Kunmi's Entry

Ibi seemed and looked better today. I wished that he would stay home. I later called Dr. Najarian to share my concern and he felt that if Ibi was up to it, I should let him. He said work provides a necessary distraction from the effects of the medication. What he said made sense and appeased my mind, but I'll still continue to suggest that Ibi stay home and hope that it sinks in one day.

FRIDAY, FEBRUARY 10

Ibi's Entry

I decided to take the day off from work. It was nice to be home and not worrying about work's problems or giving directions. I took my medication and vitamins in the morning. I laid in bed most of the day. I later went out at around three p.m.

My doctor called to inform me about my AIDS test and I was scared. He said it was negative. What a relief! The last thing I need to hear right now is about another complication.

I went to my old workplace payroll office to request my W-2 form for my tax return. I was told they would mail it to me. Then I went to the store to pay for the gas stove we purchased for our tenant and to pick Sayo up at school.

We came home and had dinner. I had an appointment with Kunmi's brother at seven p.m. to setup a UNIX network and left around 6:30 p.m. He was late. I had to wait until his business partner showed up. I was there until ten p.m. Kunmi came to join us there. Later I came home and took my medication, then went to bed.

	Breakfast	Lunch	Dinner
	Quaker Oats	Pork chops, squash and cornbread	Noodles and turkey, cranberry juice
Medications	600 mg of Ribavirin		600 mg of Ribavirin
Vitamins	500 mg of C, 400IU of E, Multi-Vitamin		500 mg of C

Kunmi's Entry

I can't believe that Ibi stayed home today. He could actually get the rest that he desperately needed without me and Sayo to bother him. I checked the refrigerator to make sure there was food for lunch and there was.

I decided to go to M.T. to force them to cut the meeting short because not only does Ibi need his rest, it was way past Sayo's bedtime. As soon as I got there, I gave them a "wrap it up" look, everyone understood and we were on our way home. Sayo barely made it to my car before falling asleep. I drove behind Ibi for safety. Ibi was so exhausted that he slept with his shoes on.

I wonder if there are any repercussions with the medications for staying up late and putting so much stress on the body.

Saturday, February 11

Ibi's Entry

I woke up and called the delivery guys about the gas stove. I was told that the delivery time will be between eleven a.m. and three p.m. I called the plumbing company to find out who would connect the gas stove. The lady told me she would get back to me soon.

I ate breakfast, took my three vitamins and waited for the contractors to show up by two p.m. I called the store and the delivery company to tell them that if my appliance is late, I would refer to them any late charges by the plumber for having to wait for their company. The delivery guys arrived minutes before three p.m. and the plumbing guy was still around to connect the gas range. There were no late charges.

I was supposed to meet M.T. at four p.m. I called him and he said he was not going to make the appointment. I kept on reading about the Internet because I was trying to get involved in the World Wide Web. I ate about three plates of rice before the afternoon, then Kunmi and I went to the store to do some shopping. I took my injection, Ribavirin and vitamins, before I left home. I felt depressed. While we were grocery shopping, I thought cooking something special for myself would help. The idea of roasting a duck appealed to me, so we bought one.

I was a little tired when we got back. I ate dinner, I watched TV for a little while, then went to sleep.

	Breakfast	Lunch	Dinner
	Oat bran and Cornflakes cereals	Three plates of rice with turkey stew	Lots of ice cream and cake
Medications	600 mg of Ribavirin		.2cc Interferon, 600 mg of Ribavirin
Vitamins	500 mg of C, 400IU of E, Multi-Vitamin		500 mg of C

Kunmi's Entry

Ibi stayed with Sayo until I got back from school. M.J. and Cheryl asked Sayo to spend the day and weekend. Cheryl and I work for the same software company. The company has a daycare in which Sayo and MJ were in the same pre-school class, and they've been friends since. They came in from Andover, Massachusetts, a thirty-mile distance, to get Sayo. As soon as they left, Ibi and I went grocery shopping until 8:30 p.m. He was exhausted. He took his injection and went straight to bed.

SUNDAY, FEBRUARY 12

Ibi's Entry

I woke up today with a pain in my throat, as if I am coming down with a cold. I tried to stay longer in bed before I took my medicine. Our gas boiler shut off. Since we have a maintenance agreement with the gas company, I called them to fix the problem. I felt depressed, but the good thing is that the depression was focused on my job. I have started to really dislike my job.

I seasoned and roasted a whole duck in the oven for lunch. I took my medications, and had hot chocolate about four times today. I watched TV to try to relax, but my mind kept returning to my work. I will be supervising a work-study student tomorrow and I'm not sure how to plan her work load.

	Breakfast	Lunch	Dinner
	Oat bran cereal with hot chocolate	Roasted duck, hot chocolate	Nigerian Cuisine - Rice, spinach with fish stew
Medications	600 mg of Ribavirin		600 mg of Ribavirin
Vitamins	500 mg of C, 400IU of E, Multi-Vitamin		500 mg of C

Kunmi's Entry

The house was freezing today. Sayo's room is usually the warmest in the house, but it was cold. I turned the heat up to eighty-five degrees and thirty minutes later there was no sign of the radiators warming up. I noticed the boiler was not working at ten a.m. and called the gas company. They did not show up until five p.m. So we huddled together with all the blankets in the house on the dining room floor. I turned the oven on and it warmed up the kitchen and dining room.

Ibi filled the draft in the living room with the sealants we bought from the hardware store. He got very tired and feverish soon after, so I finished it.

I went to pick Sayo up in Andover and returned at 6:30 p.m. Ibi was in the basement changing the water from the boilers. He said the gas person said the pilot light was out.

MONDAY, FEBRUARY 13

Ibi's Entry

I felt very exhausted when I woke up. At work, I showed the work-study student some of her responsibilities. I had a sore throat, so I called my doctor to find out if I could take lozenges. He said I could and if the pain gets stronger, I could take Tylenol.

I went to Sayo's school to pick him up. He said he behaved in school. We had dinner. I took my injection, Ribavirin and vitamins. I did some work around the house then lay down in bed and went to sleep.

	Breakfast	Lunch	Dinner
	Fish sandwich and hot chocolate	Chicken noodle soup	Turkey soup with bread
Medications	600 mg of Ribavirin		.2cc Interferon 600 mg of Ribavirin
Vitamins	500 mg of C, 400IU of E, Multi-Vitamin		500 mg of C

Kunmi's Entry

Ibi looked very tired and I advised him to stay home, but he didn't.

Ibi picked Sayo from school and I took the opportunity to do the grocery shopping at a nearby store. I got home, fed the boys, and went off to school. Ibi was snoring when I got back. I woke him up because I couldn't sleep and needed some company. He does it to me all the time.

TUESDAY, FEBRUARY 14, 1995

Ibi's Entry

I woke up with a sore throat and also felt exhausted. I took my morning medicine, and I felt very tired throughout the day. I did not feel any better after lunch. I should have stayed home today.

I came home and had dinner. I fixed Sayo's Nintendo and took my second set of medicine for the day. Then I went to bed to rest. I woke up at 10:40 p.m. and had some hot chocolate.

	Breakfast	Lunch	Dinner
	English muffin and hot chocolate	Fish dinner, an orange, grapes and yogurt	Nigerian Cuisine - Eba, spinach and turkey stew, 10 p.m. - hot chocolate and an english muffin
Medications	600 mg of Ribavirin		.2cc Interferon, 600 mg of Ribavirin
Vitamins	500 mg of C, 400IU of E, Multi-Vitamin		500 mg of C

Kunmi's Entry

Ibi looked terrible this morning, the worst that I had seen him since the treatment began. I told him to stay home, but he didn't. It suddenly dawned on me that he may fear being alone in the house. I was not sure how to initiate the conversation on fear, so I said nothing.

I went to an Internet class, then picked Sayo up from school. Ibi did not get home until six p.m. I was angry with him because my class started at 5:45 p.m. Apparently, he stopped on his way home to pick up Interferon Alfa from the pharmacy, which didn't have to be done today, because he still had two to three more treatments in the existing bottle.

I didn't appreciate him making me late for class and left angrily. He ignored me as if he had no idea why I was angry. I think Ibi is having problems concentrating due to the medication. He also looked disoriented.

WEDNESDAY, FEBRUARY 15

Ibi's Entry

I woke up with a sore throat and my mouth was dry. I took my medication with breakfast. I went to see my doctor around 5:30 p.m. He took my blood for my weekly tests. He said my hematocrit (the ratio of cells to a given volume of blood) was low and that he would draw some blood to reduce my iron level. I am starting to get used to going there every Wednesday. He told me he would be traveling to Florida for vacation, and he had made arrangements for me to see someone at Mt. Auburn Hospital. He scheduled me for the following Wednesday.

	Breakfast	Lunch	Dinner
	Hot chocolate and an English muffin	Frozen dinner - Fish, an apple, yogurt, grapes and an orange	Seasoned lamb and cabbage
Medications	600 mg of Ribavirin		600 mg of Ribavirin
Vitamins	500 mg of C, 400IU of E, Multi-Vitamin		500 mg of C

Kunmi's Entry

Roberta, my girlfriend, picked up Sayo from school because Ibi had to meet Dr. Najarian and I don't feel Sayo should go with him to the appointment. I think it is overwhelming for Ibi to have Sayo there and distracting for Dr. Najarian.

I picked up Sayo from Roberta's after my class and got home at 10:15 p.m. Ibi was fast asleep. I put the sleeping Sayo to bed and crashed into bed myself.

THURSDAY, FEBRUARY 16

Ibi's Entry

I had a slight pain in my throat today. It was a very busy day at work. When I got home in the evening, I lay down in bed to get some rest and also did some reading in the process. I took my medication and vitamins. I drank a lot of water because my throat was dry. I kept going to the bathroom every fifteen to twenty minutes.

	Breakfast	Lunch	Dinner
	Hot chocolate and an English muffin	Frozen dinner - Sirloin steak, apple, and yogurt	Ravioli
Medications	600 mg of Ribavirin		.2cc Interferon, 600 mg of Ribavirin
Vitamins	500 mg of C, 400IU of E, Multi-Vitamin		500 mg of C

Kunmi's Entry

Ibi complained about being tired, but he wouldn't stay home. I was becoming very upset, but I tried not to show it. I went to a seminar at a major networking company. Since Ibi was fed up with his current job, and job hunting, I submitted his resume to the human resource office while I was there.

I went alone to Boston City Hospital to visit Jasmine, one of Sayo's classmates. She is a five year old girl who has water in her brain that could not be drained out. She was on life support and heavily medicated but quite alert. Jasmine's mother was not there and the nurses could not let me in the room. It took two hours to locate her mother. I had come to visit the girl and refused to leave until I had done just that. Her mother spoke to me on the phone, gave her okay and the nurses let me into the room.

It was a pathetic sight and I felt it may have been better if I hadn't seen her. She seemed upset, making sounds and tears came out of her eyes. I started crying too. I stroked her hand and told her Sayo said hello, and she would be okay. What a liar I was! From what I heard of the diagnosis, she has a one percent chance or less of recovery of speech or any other bodily function.

Friday, February 17

Ibi's Entry

I woke up a little tired. I took my medication. Things were very busy at work today. After I had lunch, I felt really tired. I felt like lying down in my office and going to sleep. Because of my concern for my responsibilities, I could not take the day off. I feel very responsible for the improvements we are making to the software we are developing for our environmental program. I had to show the student helping with the data entry what to do so that we could start using the Information System. After about two hours, I felt a little stronger and finished my day at work. I got out at about 5:50 p.m. and went to Sayo's school for a pot luck event. We had dinner there.

I saw a friend and his son at the pot luck. [For privacy, their names have been left out.] He informed me about his wife's problems with her pregnancy. He told me she was admitted into the hospital. Kunmi and I decided to keep their son so that he could spend time with his wife in the hospital. We visited the wife at the hospital that night. We came home, and I was very tired so I went to bed. I took my second round of medication at 10:15 p.m. when I came home.

	Breakfast	Lunch	Dinner
	Grapefruit juice, bread and hot chocolate	Rice and turkey stew	Barbecue fried chicken with garden salad, coleslaw, bread rolls and cornbread, punch and cake
Medications	600 mg of Ribavirin		600 mg of Ribavirin
Vitamins	500 mg of C, 400IU of E, Multi-Vitamin		500 mg of C

Kunmi's Entry

Ibi complained about being tired when I called him in the afternoon. I told him to come home, but he said he had to show the work study girl her assignment. He called at 5:30 p.m. to say he had been delayed at work and came home after six p.m.

Ibi ate a lot at the pot luck dinner. He looked exhausted.

SATURDAY, FEBRUARY 18

Ibi's Entry

I woke feeling well rested. Sayo and our guest woke me up asking for their breakfast. I made our guest an egg sandwich and Sayo, beefaroni. I had a small breakfast then lay back in bed to rest my mind and watch TV.

I used watching TV to deal with any likelihood of depression from the medication. I watch mostly the cable news channels which is quite informative and interesting. It has worked so far. I get so depressed that the thought of committing suicide has occurred to me. Once in a while, I have flashes of this idea and I immediately tell myself that I must be out of my mind. There is so much to live for. I need to live for my country, brothers and sisters and to help people unite their families.

I stayed in bed most of the day trying to rest my mind. Later in the day, we went grocery shopping. I took my injection before we went shopping and also my second round of medication. I came back home and had dinner. I felt really tired, couldn't concentrate and therefore could not study the UNIX administration book, so I went and lay in bed. I also had trouble falling asleep.

	Breakfast	Lunch	Dinner
	Two slices of bread and hot chocolate	Turkey Soup	Lamb and cabbage, ice cream
Medications	600 mg of Ribavirin		.2cc Interferon, 600 mg of Ribavirin
Vitamins	500 mg of C, 400IU of E, Multi-Vitamin		500 mg of C

Kunmi's Entry

I went to school at 8:30 a.m. and Ibi stayed with the boys. After class, I went to see my friend whose son we have for the weekend, at the hospital. She gave me a change of clothes for her son.

I came home and found the boys in the park. Ibi was having fun playing ball with the boys. I picked them up to do grocery. The boys were exhausted and asleep by the time I drove home from the store. Ibi woke up as soon as I parked the car.

Sunday, February 19, 1995

Ibi's Entry

I woke up well rested. It seems that any time I eat, I get really tired and want to sleep again. I felt better after sleeping a while. Then I took my first round of medication for the morning. I did some work around the house, cleaned the bathroom, did laundry. I got really tired again and went to bed. I stayed there most of the day.

Our friend came over and told us his wife lost her baby early that morning. He was quite depressed. We talked for a while. I tried to console him, I felt depressed myself. I felt that mine can be stopped if I discontinued my medication, but his is beyond his control. I shared with him my experience of losing my mother to breast cancer in 1991. That depressed me even more because I was extremely close to my mother and I still miss her terribly.

As soon as he left, I immediately went back to bed. Staying in bed is helping me balance my thoughts. More than ever, I needed to focus on something else, so I put on the TV as I lay there. I got up and took my second round of medication at around 5:30 p.m. and went back to bed. I fed the kids pizza at night and I had some too. Our guest was crying for his mommy, so I told him and Sayo to watch TV with me in the bedroom.

It was a good idea to have them in the bedroom. I didn't have to worry about what they were doing, meaning that I did not have to get out of bed. It was also a desperately needed distraction because they were asking questions about the nature program we were watching, and I had to answer. They both went to sleep and so did I.

	Breakfast	Lunch	Dinner
	Oat Bran cereal and hot chocolate	Beef cooked with mushrooms, red pepper, onion and cabbage	Pizza
Medications	600 mg of Ribavirin		600 mg of Ribavirin
Vitamins	500 mg of C, 400IU of E, Multi-Vitamin		500 mg of C

Kunmi's Entry

Ibi looked and still seemed exhausted. He ate and went back to bed. I was sad to hear that our friend lost her baby.

MONDAY, FEBRUARY 20

Ibi's Entry

I woke up feeling very good. The problem seems to be my tiredness. I just get tired all of a sudden and after a while, I feel better, full of energy. I ate pizza for breakfast and went back to bed. After a while, I got up to do the laundry. I took my first round of medication before doing this.

To my surprise, all the clothes came out right. I was so proud of myself and it felt good. I did three more loads and left one in the washer to soak for a day.

We went for our tax return appointment. We missed the lady, so we stopped to do some shopping. We also stopped by the house of the friend who just got back from the hospital. We spent about thirty minutes there and came back home. I folded some laundry. Later I went to bed to get some rest. I felt powerless because I always get tired easily.

It was a nice day overall, but I started feeling depressed about going to work tomorrow. I ironed my clothes, then I took my injection and my second round of medication around 5:30 p.m.

	Breakfast	Lunch	Dinner
	Pizza, hot chocolate with milk	Skipped lunch	Chicken and rice with curry and a biscuit
Medications	600 mg of Ribavirin		.2cc Interferon, 600 mg of Ribavirin
Vitamins	500 mg of C, 400IU of E, Multi-Vitamin		500 mg of C

Kunmi's Entry

Ibi brought work home and was doing it when I got home. He did three loads of laundry and the whites he soaked yesterday. He ate dinner and had a good appetite. I went to bed late and couldn't sleep until after midnight.

TUESDAY, FEBRUARY 21

Ibi's Entry

I woke up feeling a little bit of pain in both of my arm joints. It was something I could ignore and still go about my normal work schedule. I had breakfast while my wife packed lunch. I took my first round of medication and set out to work.

I had a meeting with my manager to update him on what was happening with the computer database setup. I went through the day without any problems, but when I got home I felt very tired so I went to sleep. I woke up around 11:30 p.m. to do my office work. I wrote my memo around 1:30 a.m. and went back to sleep shortly after.

	Breakfast	Lunch	Dinner
	Hot chocolate	Rice with glazed chicken and grapes	Spaghetti and meatballs
Medications	600 mg of Ribavirin		600 mg of Ribavirin
Vitamins	500 mg of C, 400IU of E, Multi-Vitamin		500 mg of C

Kunmi's Entry

I got up from bed at 7:45 a.m. and everything seemed normal. I dropped off and picked Sayo up from school. I took Sayo to a fast food restaurant on the way home, he was happy. We got home at six p.m. and Ibi was already home and sound asleep. He looked exhausted. He woke up to work on an office project. I went to bed about 12 a.m., and he was still working on it.

WEDNESDAY, FEBRUARY 22

Ibi's Entry

I woke up in good health, even though I did not get to bed until three a.m. I had breakfast and took my morning round of medication. Everything was okay at work.

I left work pretending that I was sick because I had an appointment at Mt. Auburn Hospital, which Dr. Najarian scheduled for me before going on vacation. I was not comfortable revealing my Hepatitis infection to my co-workers because I was not sure how they would react. I knew that the only person at risk of infection were my wife and son. If there were a remote chance of infecting someone at work, I would tell them and stay home, but that is not the case. Moreover, work helps me pass the time quickly.

They took one pint of blood and it took about an hour. At the hospital, the guy that attended to me was from Panama. He knows my doctor and said he is a very intelligent man and I am lucky to have him take care of me. I had some cranberry juice while I was there.

I came home and went directly to bed. I was very tired. I woke up around 8:30 p.m. and had dinner. Then I took my second round of medication. I wrote my memo and watched some T.V. I also did some laundry.

	Breakfast	Lunch	Dinner
	Turkey with cheese sandwich, hot chocolate	Turkey burger	Rice and chicken, cranberry juice
Medications	600 mg of Ribavirin		600 mg of Ribavirin
Vitamins	500 mg of C, 400IU of E, Multi-Vitamin		500 mg of C

Kunmi's Entry

Ibi is having his blood drawn at Mount Auburn because Dr. Najarian is on vacation in Florida. He said he felt dizzy afterward and was as tired as usual. I asked who was better at drawing the blood and he said the hospital was. I suggested that he may want to suggest to Dr. Najarian to let him have the blood drawn at the hospital instead. He said that he prefers that Dr. Najarian continue as he has.

THURSDAY, FEBRUARY 23

Ibi's Entry

I woke up in good condition. I ironed my shirt and tie for work and took a bath, like I do every morning. I also took the first round of medication. Then I had breakfast and left home for work. It was a very busy day.

I had a late lunch around three p.m. I left work around 5:10 p.m. to pick Sayo up from school. We had dinner and I took my injection and my second round of medication.

Dr. Najarian will return from vacation on Friday. I can't wait to hear the results of my blood test. I stayed in bed to watch TV and also to think about my future. The current results of the treatment are not encouraging. Dr. Najarian and Kunmi are hopeful that the treatment will be successful. I am not so confident. I deal with the present and can't see beyond how I currently feel. I would like to be cured and go on to live a normal and stress-free life. I would like to get married and have many healthy children. I would like to have a job that I am happy to go to every morning. I would like many great things in my future.....I fell asleep.

	Breakfast	Lunch	Dinner
	Hot chocolate, three slices of bread	Tuna sandwich	Pizza and bread sticks
Medications	600 mg of Ribavirin		.2cc Interferon 600 mg of Ribavirin
Vitamins	500 mg of C, 400IU of E, Multi-Vitamin		500 mg of C

Kunmi's Entry

Ibi still looked tired. Again, I tried to convince him to stay home, but he didn't. My vacation is over today, so off to work I go. Ibi did more laundry in the evening. I wondered what had gotten into him. He is actually doing a good job. The clothes come out clean.

FRIDAY, FEBRUARY 24

Ibi's Entry

I woke up in good health, but I was tired. I thought about calling in sick. I did my morning exercises, then went back to sleep. Later I woke up, had breakfast, took my first round of medication and went to work. I left home late and got to work around 11:30 a.m. I had a very busy day. I came home and took my second round of medication. I did not really have an appetite and I went to bed very early.

	Breakfast	Lunch	Dinner
	Quaker Oats, Hot chocolate	Noodle soup	Can of corn
Medications	600 mg of Ribavirin		600 mg of Ribavirin
Vitamins	500 mg of C, 400IU of E, Multi-Vitamin		500 mg of C

Kunmi's Entry

I managed to get Ibi to sleep in by disabling the alarm, which made him late for work. Sayo also got to school late. He was so happy that we let him sleep longer and watch a little T.V. before going to school. After school, he went with Roberta to see a play "Winnie the Pooh" at Wheelock College in Boston, so Ibi got a break and time to rest after work. He was in bed when I came in with Sayo at 9:30 p.m.

Saturday, February 25

Ibi's Entry

I woke up very tired. I did some work in the kitchen before I went back to bed to get more rest. Kunmi went to school and Sayo stayed home with me.

I called my father in Nigeria to see how he was doing and to update him on my health. There really was no good news to convey. My brother, Layemi, also called from London to see how I was doing. Later, my eldest brother, Dr. Oluwole Oluleye, called from Nigeria. He was having a birthday party for his son Dayo, today but was thinking of me. All the immediate family were there. It was a good opportunity to speak with everyone. I talked with my sisters, nieces and nephews.

I had an appointment to meet Kunmi's brother M.T. to help me set up my computer with Linux, a UNIX software. I took my second round of medication around four p.m. before I left home. It took us about six hours to install. I got home around 11:50 p.m. and Kunmi had ordered Chinese food. I ate that before going to bed. I took my injection at midnight and went to bed.

	Breakfast	Lunch	Dinner
	Hot chocolate	Pizza	Chinese food
Medications	600 mg of Ribavirin		.2cc Interferon, 600 mg of Ribavirin
Vitamins	500 mg of C, 400IU of E, Multi-Vitamin		500 mg of C

Kunmi's Entry

I went to school at 8:30 a.m. as usual and got home at 2:30 p.m. to find Ibi cooking. I have neglected my household chores for the past few weeks and must catch up this week. He filled the dishwasher with dirty dishes and turned it on, and did more laundry.

SUNDAY, FEBRUARY 26

Ibi's Entry

I took my first round of medication after a late breakfast. I cleaned the kitchen, watched some TV, and slept. I set up the computer at home but had some problems using the DOS operating system. I learned more UNIX commands. I was on it till about eleven p.m.

I planned the staff budget for work. I resumed watching TV for some time, then later took my second round of medication and went to bed.

	Breakfast	Lunch	Dinner
	Chinese food	Skipped lunch	Nigerian Cuisine - Eba, turkey and apon stew
Medications	600 mg of Ribavirin		600 mg of Ribavirin
Vitamins	500 mg of C, 400IU of E, Multi-Vitamin		500 mg of C

Kunmi's Entry

Ibi washed all the dishes, pots in the sink and ran the dishwasher. He ate Chinese food for breakfast and fed Sayo the same.

He was excited about the UNIX on the computer and sat with it all afternoon. Sayo and I went to an indoor playhouse at three p.m. and came back at seven p.m. Ibi was in bed reading. I cooked and we ate.

MONDAY, FEBRUARY 27

Ibi's Entry

I woke up in good health. I have been trying to keep very busy so that I don't get depressed. I took my first round of medication in the morning and went to work. I also had some breakfast. I tried to keep myself very busy.

I called my doctor to get the results of my blood test. He told me the liver enzymes were about the same as the last time and that my white counts were low. He told me he was going to introduce a hormone into my medication to boost my white count. I did not feel good about this. I told myself that as long as I have energy and feel somewhat healthy, life goes on. If I have to add another medication to cure this illness, I have no choice but to cope with it.

I came home after I picked Sayo up from school. Then I took my injection and my second round of medication. I learned more UNIX commands on the computer before I went to bed.

	Breakfast	Lunch	Dinner
	Hot chocolate with milk	Roasted turkey and vegetables	Sausage, onion and pepper pizza
Medications	600 mg of Ribavirin		.2cc Interferon, 600 mg of Ribavirin
Vitamins	500 mg of C, 400IU of E, Multi-Vitamin		500 mg of C

Kunmi's Entry

Today was the first day of fasting for me. In observance of lent, fasting does not really start until Wednesday, known as Ash Wednesday. I thought I should use today and tomorrow as practice days. It is said that fasting during lent or at any other time is a cleansing method and a better time to ask the higher power for one's heart's desire.

I got home at 8:30 p.m., and Ibi was on the computer playing with UNIX. I gave him the UNIX administration guide I had borrowed from a girl at work. He was very happy, took the book and went to bed reading it until ten p.m.

Tuesday, February 28

Ibi's Entry

I woke up tired. I ate breakfast and took my first round of medication before leaving for work. I was very busy at work which kept me from getting depressed. This was something I taught myself after I lost my mum. To deal with her loss, I had to keep myself very busy so that I wouldn't think about the pain. She was very close and dear to me.

I came home very tired and took my second round of medication. I called my doctor earlier in the day to find out about the Ferritin level (iron) in my liver. He said the results were not good, it was high. He said the disease might be causing this problem and he is going to do other tests on me. He also explained that my low white counts may be naturally low. I was angry at the news. It's been almost six weeks since I started the treatment, and it seemed that things are getting worse instead of better. My stomach looked blotted. Doing the morning exercise doesn't really seem to help because my liver is still swollen which is what happens to the stomach of the infected

Hepatitis victim. It is quite frustrating to have no control over one's condition.

I felt really tired and rested in bed for about two hours when I got home. I reflected back on the news I got from Dr. Najarian and felt that as gloomy as the situation looks, I felt lucky to have the opportunity to undergo this combination treatment, because I have a chance to cure this disease. I may not have to live with it and treat the symptoms like millions of others. I would rather cure it once and for all. I'll try to remain open and hear other suggestions Dr. Najarian may have.

	Breakfast	Lunch	Dinner
	Hot chocolate and bread	Steak and cheese sub	Rice and fish stew
Medications	600 mg of Ribavirin		600 mg of Ribavirin
Vitamins	500 mg of C, 400IU of E, Multi-Vitamin		500 mg of C

Kunmi's Entry

Second day of fasting and I did it again. It was an extremely slippery day. The roads were treacherous but I still had to go to work. Sayo's school was closed, so I took him to work with me. He sat in my cubicle and wandered around a bit. Overall, he behaved.

Ibi went to work also. He looked extremely depressed. He barely says anything and I am really worried. I asked how he was doing and he nodded fine. I felt that I should read his journal to find out what's going on with him. I didn't because we both made a promise not to read each other's journal until the treatment is over.

Chapter Six

The Lord is my sherperd
I shall not want.

Wednesday, March 1

Ibi's Entry

I woke up in good condition. I did not feel any headaches or pains. I took my first round of medication in the morning with some orange juice. I tried to keep myself very busy at work. I was supposed to move my office to the second floor the next day, so I packed some of my belongings and did some of my routine work.

On visiting my doctor that evening, he told me that my blood count was low and that he would show me how to use a hormone to help boost my white cell count to help fight the disease. My doctor believes that the higher white count there is to fight the disease, the weaker the virus will be. This seemed to be a very simple theory that when you attack an enemy with bombs for days without them having enough time to recuperate, the enemy gets weaker and won't have enough strength to fight back. That was our strategy for fighting the disease. It seems that the virus is able protect itself from Interferon Alfa-2b and Ribavirin. If a third medication is introduced, the virus now has three enemies to deal with. Our hope is that it cannot fight off all three medications at the same time, and therefore will weaken.

Dr. Najarian gave me the prescription for the white blood count booster (hormone). As usual, his wife went upstairs to cook some soup. She made sure I ate some so I would gain some energy. While I was at their house, I was introduced to her brother. This was the brother that was discussed in Chapter Three whom Dr. Najarian cured of disease of the polys. I finished the soup, and we all sat down and talked for a while.

I stopped by the pharmacy to request the hormone and I was told to pick it up the next day. My fiancée was already waiting for me at home. I took my second round of medication and studied more UNIX administration before going to bed.

	Breakfast	Lunch	Dinner
	Orange juice	Big bowl of rice and about three chunks of turkey meat	Wheat soup
Medications	600 mg of Ribavirin		600 mg of Ribavirin
Vitamins	500 mg of C, 400IU of E, Multi-Vitamin		500 mg of C

Kunmi's Entry

Official fasting day — Ash Wednesday.

I am quite prepared to fast for the next forty days. This is the second year that I will be doing this. My fasting is to give up all food and drink from midnight to six p.m. I did it again today. Only 39 days to go. Today's fasting was easy because I got a two-day practice start. I didn't even realize it was six p.m. and time to eat. Last year, during fasting I prayed to meet a man who would respect and love me and also my child. I feel that prayer was answered that year when Ibi said he wanted a serious relationship.

My prayer for this year is that Ibi will be cured, that God will continue to bless my life and my child, that I finish my MBA, CNE and Lotus Notes certification by the end of the year and that God keep me, Sayo and Ibi safe and healthy and give us peace. I ask the same prayer for both of our families.

There is talk of Ibi having an MRI of the liver performed. Ibi seemed unconcerned about it. I asked if he had been through the procedure before and he had not. I had an MRI performed a few years earlier and felt like sharing the experience, but he did not seem interested, so I did not discuss it. I didn't know if the MRI was a definite event or still in discussion between him and Dr. Najarian. I know that he wouldn't have one done without telling me, so I need to be patient until he is ready to talk about it.

THURSDAY, MARCH 2

Ibi's Entry

I woke up feeling very well and energized for the day. I had a busy day at work. I helped the movers who were relocating my office to another place in the building. I also lifted fifteen to twenty-five pounds of lead bricks over a distance of more than 800 meters. These bricks are used for shielding radioactive materials. I had to come up with an estimate for the fiscal year budget for the radiation safety program I manage. This was due by 12 noon the following day, so I worked on that for the later part of the afternoon. At the end of the day, I was really tired.

I called my doctor to confirm the appointment for my liver MRI, to check for excess iron. My doctor scheduled the appointment for tomorrow but had to change it to Monday, the following week, at seven a.m.

I took my second round of medication for the day as well as the injection. I did some studying on UNIX administration and went to bed.

	Breakfast	Lunch	Dinner
	Quaker Oats	Rice and stew	Rice and stew
Medications	600 mg of Ribavirin		.2cc Interferon, 600 mg of Ribavirin
Vitamins	500 mg of C, 400IU of E, Multi-Vitamin		500 mg of C

Kunmi's Entry

Ibi started the day out okay, but he ended up being cranky. He must have had a bad day at work. He is tired of his director asking for things at the last minute. I wondered whether he is more sensitive to work situations because of the thought of having an MRI done.

I retrieved the message on the answering machine while at work, and found that Dr. Najarian called to schedule the MRI. I was surprised, I didn't realize that Ibi was definitely having one performed, so I called Dr. Najarian.

The white blood count is low, and iron is still high. Enzyme level is high and not changing much. The prescribed hormone to raise the white cell count has effected no change.

That night at home, Ibi was disappointed about the progress of the treatment so far. I was still hopeful. I hugged him to comfort and reassure him. We talked about his upcoming MRI and he was worried about not only the process, but also the result. I told him about my experience with the MRI, which is a machine that takes pictures of one's internal organs. The machine is usually the shape of a tube with an alarm that one can pull, if one needs to come out at any time for any reason. This may be a difficult procedure for someone who is claustrophobic.

I was put in a full-body MRI machine, even though I had a head scan done. My whole body was in this enclosed tube and I was scared. However, there are many different full and half-body types of equipment, depending on which part of the body is being examined and who is performing the MRI. A friend who recently had an MRI of the head performed at an MRI specialized center, was place in a half-body unit, which has a mirror inside the tube to allow her see the MRI technician. Because it was a half-body unit, she could move her legs and therefore did not feel so enclosed. An MRI center usually has the most recent and more user-friendly equipment. Some units are capable of playing music, giving one the choice of listening to the radio or favorite tape.

I asked if he is claustrophobic and he said he isn't. He felt better.

Friday, March 3

Ibi's Entry

I made sure I took my first round of medication before I left home. I left for work early, feeling a little tired. I was very busy with my supervisor trying to come up with the best budget for our group. I could not wait to get home because I was so tired. I stopped by the pharmacy to pick up the hormone medication. When I got home, I took my medication and hormone. The days I inject the hormone will vary depending on the result of the last blood test.

	Breakfast	Lunch	Dinner
	Quaker Oats	Tuna sandwich	Nigerian cuisine - Amala, turkey and spinach stew
Medications	600 mg of Ribavirin		.2cc Interferon, 600 mg of Ribavirin, 1ml white count booster hormone
Vitamins	500 mg of C, 400IU of E, Multi-Vitamin		500 mg of C

Kunmi's Entry

Ibi seemed to be in an okay mood. He picked Sayo up from school and sent him to bed early because he misbehaved in class. Ibi started taking his new hormone and seemed really down that he needs to add another medication. He was in bed, but awake when I got home. We talked about his new hormone and he did not feel any additional side effect from it. He said that even though he was exhausted, he has trouble falling asleep. We talked about other stuff and he finally dozed off.

SATURDAY, MARCH 4

Ibi's Entry

I woke up feeling fine; not going to work today contributed to the great feeling. I cleaned the house and had some soup that my doctor's wife made for me. Then I took my morning round of medication and did more cleaning. I took Kunmi's car to the garage to get her tire fixed. I came home and took a bath and I fixed the B drive on my computer. I slept for about forty-five minutes because I was really tired.

Kunmi came home and we went to Attleboro which is near the state of Rhode Island, to play the power-ball lottery. On the way home, we stopped by to pick up my friend who lost the baby and her son to spend the night. We all went to a Thai restaurant in Cambridge to have dinner and came home.

When we got home I took my medication. After a while I started feeling achy and feverish, which indicates that my medication is working. I have not felt this way in a while. This might be why the enzyme levels for my liver have not dropped that much. I think the hormone is helping me fight the disease. I tried to study UNIX, but I was too tired and went to sleep.

	Breakfast	Lunch	Dinner
	Yam soup	Yam soup	Thai food
Medications	600 mg of Ribavirin		.2cc Interferon, 600 mg of Ribavirin, 1ml white count booster hormone
Vitamins	500 mg of C, 400IU of E, Multi-Vitamin		500 mg of C

Kunmi's Entry

I dropped Sayo at my friend's house in the morning on the way to school. Later I picked Ibi up and went to play the lottery. On the way, we talked about not having to pay full price for the Hepatitis treatment. Our medical insurance covered most of it. We talked about what we would buy if we won.

We came home exhausted. Ibi collapsed in bed and the boys did the same. My friend and myself stayed up talking till four a.m. We talked about her failed pregnancy, how she felt before, during and after, and hopes for the future. We talked about relationships and ingredients for a successful one. We talked about the hepatitis treatment and its effect on Ibi, Sayo and me. We talked about children, how many, when to have them and how to raise them, and many other things.

SUNDAY, MARCH 5

Ibi's Entry

I woke up feeling achy, tired and feverish. Kunmi made a delicious breakfast for all of us. It was nice to have company. Kunmi, our friend and I sat down at the dining room table and talked for a while. I got tired and went to the bedroom to lie down with the kids. I also took my morning medication.

Throughout the day I snacked on pieces of fried goat's meat. I did not have much of an appetite throughout the day. We all went to the movies in the evening. I fell asleep in the movie theater for a while.

When we came back home, I took my second round of medication. I went to bed very early because I was tired and have my MRI very early tomorrow morning.

	Breakfast	Lunch	Dinner
	Bread, jelly and scrambled eggs with cornbeef, onion, tomatoes and pepper, curry, thyme	Goat's meat stew with rice	Goat's meat stew with Eba
Medications	600 mg of Ribavirin		600 mg of Ribavirin, 1ml white count booster hormone
Vitamins	500 mg of C, 400IU of E, Multi-Vitamin		500 mg of C

Kunmi's Entry

I woke up at 8:25 a.m. to fix breakfast for everyone. Ibi developed a fever overnight and had it for most of the day. He seemed very tired and spent a good amount of the day in bed.

Our guests went home at seven p.m. Ibi's fever was high, but he did not take Tylenol. He and Sayo went to bed before eight p.m., after he took his hormone shot. I went to bed much later.

Monday, March 6

Ibi's Entry

I woke up around 5:30 a.m. to get ready for my MRI appointment at 6:30 a.m. I was anxious. I did not eat anything because I was instructed not to prior to the procedure, but Kunmi made me two egg sandwiches to eat after the MRI.

I arrived at the hospital a few minutes before 6:30 a.m. The MRI technician who will be taking the pictures went over the procedure, showed me the machine and asked if I had any questions. The amount of time it will take depends on the number of pictures that need to be taken and how much imagery need to be captured.

I was to be injected with a liquid called Gadolinium, a contract agent used during the scan. The liquid makes the iron in my liver show in the pictures. She explained that the side effects were headaches, nausea and vomitting. I signed the consent form and was injected with the Gadolinium.

No jewelry is allowed in machine, so I removed my jewelry. I had the option of ear plugs or music, to block the drumming noise the machine makes when taking pictures. I chose the music.

I lay on a table which was pulled into the MRI machine when the technician pushed a button on the side of the machine. My entire body was in the tube. It was an interesting experience because it felt like being in a coffin. Surprisingly, I was calm. I left the hospital at 7:55 a.m. I ate the egg sandwiches.

Even though I was very busy at work, I needed a change of scenery and came home for lunch. It was good. I rushed home after work. I changed the water in my turtles' tank.

I took my second round of medication and injection. I did some studying on UNIX. Kunmi and I also did our monthly expense accounting. This took a while. As soon as it was done, we went to bed.

	Breakfast	Lunch	Dinner
	Two egg sandwiches with cheese on English muffin, hot chocolate	Eba and turkey stew	Spaghetti and meatballs with mixed vegetables
Medications	Gadolinium, 600 mg of Ribavirin		.2cc Interferon, 600 mg of Ribavirin
Vitamins	500 mg of C, 400IU of E, Multi-Vitamin		500 mg of C

Kunmi's Entry

Ibi went to his MRI. He seemed quite calm. I asked him if he wanted me to come, and he bluntly refused. We discussed the procedure while I made him take-away breakfast. I gave him the usual hug and kiss, and he left in good spirits. In the evening, we talked about how the MRI went. He joked about the tube and its similarity to a coffin, and that he hopes that it's not the prelude of things to come.

I asked why he didn't mention that he was having an MRI done as soon as Dr. Najarian told him, and he said that he did not want to make it a major event. I told him that I felt left out and asked if there were other things he was keeping from me and he said no. I made him promise to always give me updates on his treatment as soon as he gets them. He is becoming more difficult to reach. He keeps distancing himself and I have to constantly stay tuned into him whether he likes it or not.

TUESDAY, MARCH 7

Ibi's Entry

I woke up feeling a little feverish and achy. I had some cereal for breakfast and I took my morning medication. I had a problem with a guy I work with. He feels that he is smarter and doesn't understand why people respect and respond to me more. He's always trying to prove that he is better than me. Today, he was so rude to me that I informed my director. I was very hungry and grateful for the perfect timing of the apples a friend at work, Lin, gave me. I ate two of them in addition to lunch. I left work at five p.m. to pick Sayo up from school.

He is a little confused as to when he is bad. He was not listening again to the teacher's instructions. The teacher's threatening to call Kunmi to report him, did not change his behavior. I need to discuss how he is doing in school with his teacher. We came home, and I gave him dinner, but first we ate the cashew nuts on the table.

I took my hormone injection and my second round of medication. Then I lay in bed and listened to the news. I also did some studying before I finally slept.

	Breakfast	Lunch	Dinner
	Oat bran cereal	Meatball sub	Rice and stew, cashew nuts
Medications	600 mg of Ribavirin		600 mg of Ribavirin, 1ml white count booster hormone
Vitamins	500 mg of C, 400IU of E, Multi-Vitamin		500 mg of C

Kunmi's Entry

Ibi called me at work to tell me that a co-worker slammed the door in his face at work after a discussion of the different opinions they had. He was slightly upset, but he handled it well. He did not say anything to the co-worker. He called his director and reported the incident. The director took this seriously and will speak with the co-worker immediately. Ibi was still upset and decided to call me to cool off. I tried to console him and told him to ignore the co-worker.

Ibi was fast asleep when I got home. He must have gone to bed early. He had a temperature overnight.

WEDNESDAY, MARCH 8

Ibi's Entry

I woke up feeling feverish and achy. I took a bath and my morning round of medication. I have not felt this feverish for a while. Maybe it is because of the hormone I am taking.

We had pizza for lunch at my staff meeting. I only ate three slices. I kept busy throughout the day.

When I visited my doctor, he told me there was no iron deposit in my liver according to the MRI test I had Monday morning. He said next week will be two months that I have been on this medication. He also informed me about DNA testing to detect if the virus is still in my system. He said if the virus is still in my system, he would introduce a third drug to help fight the disease.

When I got home in the evening, I ordered some pizza and buffalo wings for our family dinner. Kunmi and Sayo did not come home early as I expected. I was a little angry because I couldn't wait to share the good news. I took my second round of medication. I tried to study UNIX and went to bed after that.

	Breakfast	Lunch	Dinner
	Hot chocolate and bread	Three slices of pizza	Pizza and chicken wings
Medications	600 mg of Ribavirin		600 mg of Ribavirin
Vitamins	500 mg of C, 400IU of E, Multi-Vitamin		500 mg of C

Kunmi's Entry

Ibi was asleep when I got home. He had ordered two pizzas and chicken wings for us because there was minimal food in the house. I had picked up our tax returns, woke him up to see it. He was happy about his refund, but seemed a bit depressed and tired. We discussed the wedding invitation list. He cut the guest count to half and the cost to zero. I then got a lecture about money. I nagged him about not helping with the plans.

THURSDAY, MARCH 9

Ibi's Entry

I woke up feeling okay but a little feverish and achy. I ate breakfast and took my first round of medication. I went to work to keep myself busy as usual.

I called my doctor at about 1:30 p.m. to find out about the results of my blood test. He told me that my white count was very high now and that I should reduce the hormone injection to about twice a week. He said there was a strange thing in my liver enzyme level. It was higher, very high. He was expecting this to happen at the beginning of the treatment, but the enzymes stayed steady and dropped after about four weeks of treatment.

The doctor thinks there is nothing to worry about and that it may be that I have enough white blood count to fight the disease. If the virus is being destroyed, the enzyme level will rise suddenly. We are hoping the medication is working and will watch for another week to see what happens. He said to maintain the same doses for all other medications.

I came home and took my injection and second round of medication. Kunmi came home and wouldn't let me study. We talked all night about her frustration with work and school and about my high enzymes.

	Breakfast	Lunch	Dinner
	Pizza and hot chocolate	Large cheeseburger, fries and soda	Steak, baked potato and corn
Medications	600 mg of Ribavirin		.2cc Interferon, 600 mg of Ribavirin
Vitamins	500 mg of C, 400IU of E, Multi-Vitamin		500 mg of C

Kunmi's Entry

Last night's nagging worked. Ibi called to get rental prices on his tuxedo for the wedding. He told me the cost was sixty-nine dollars for the tux he wanted and for Sayo's.

Ibi got voicemail at work today and was very excited about it. He told me his budget was approved, so he's getting his network.

As I was about to go to sleep, Ibi mentioned his high liver enzymes and I tried to hide my disappointment at the news. He was frustrated because he felt that the hormone was working because of the fevers and aches which has now returned since he started taking the hormone with Interferon Alfa. He said that Dr. Najarian was also surprised at the result. Maybe he was taking too much of the hormone, but now that it has been reduced to twice a week, it might work. I told him to be patient with the new dose and in a few weeks, we should know if there's reason to panic or be upset. He agreed and we went to sleep.

FRIDAY, MARCH 10

Ibi's Entry

I woke up a little feverish and achy, but I still went to work. The day was kind of fun. I had lunch with my supervisor and we had a nice talk about the quality of my work, the budget proposal and setting up the network. Everyone at work contributed money and got a surprise marriage gift for Lin and her husband. It was nice to see everybody in a happy mood.

I am starting to feel that I will be made the network administrator for my department soon, and my job description will change. This is something I really want to do, and I am excited about it.

I picked Sayo up at school. On the way home, he showed me a loose tooth, and asked if a tooth fairy really existed. I told him she did. He was curious how much money she would give him once the tooth comes out and placed under his pillow. I told him it depends on how much she has and how good he's been.

When we got home I fed us both and I took my second round of medication and hormone injection. I felt better tonight than I did last night. I hope the hormone works with my other medications, because to go through this treatment and not be cured would have been a waste of my time, energy and emotions.

	Breakfast	Lunch	Dinner
	Quaker Oats	Turkey sub with lettuce and tomato	Lasagna
Medications	600 mg of Ribavirin		600 mg of Ribavirin, 1ml white count booster hormone
Vitamins	500 mg of C, 400IU of E, Multi-Vitamin		500 mg of C

Kunmi's Entry

Too tired and busy to make an entry.

Saturday, March 11

Ibi's Entry

I woke up tired and stayed in bed most of the day. Later, I took my first round of medication. All day I was picking at my food. I really did not have an appetite. I stayed in bed feeling achy and feverish. I believe the medication is really working. I am starting to realize that I don't have much stamina anymore. I feel very fatigued. I lay in bed watching TV most of the day, but got up to socialize with our visitors. As soon as they left, I went back to bed and watching TV.

I could not go to sleep, and my brain would not concentrate on anything, so I could not study. I soaked clothes in the washer and cleaned Kunmi's car, and then I had dinner. I took my second round of medication and injection at about 9:30 p.m. I drank hot chocolate made with milk, and that helped put me to sleep.

	Breakfast	Lunch	Dinner
	Oat bran cereal	Thai Food	Rice and stew
Medications	600 mg of Ribavirin		.2cc Interferon, 600 mg of Ribavirin
Vitamins	500 mg of C, 400IU of E, Multi-Vitamin		500 mg of C

Kunmi's Entry

My cousins, Banke and Yemisi Oluwole, my sister, Banke Tuyo and a family friend came over to visit. It seems like a full house with all the eating, drinking and talking. This was really good for Ibi in that it was a distraction from his condition. I knew that he wouldn't stay in bed with people visiting. After they all left, Ibi went back to bed, but felt restless and decided to clean my car. He had to stop because of the fever and aches. He finished it later. He was exhausted.

While Ibi was asleep, I went to our favorite Thai place and picked up some food. He was pleased to wake up to his favorite Thai dish. He ate and went right back to bed. Sayo and I spent some quiet time together talking and playing games. I refused to let him teach me Nintendo.

We talked about Ibi's treatment and how different he may have become. Sayo did not seem to mind the quietness that has now become Ibi's personality. He did notice that Ibi tires out more easily and quickly and spends more time in bed. Sayo adjusted himself to the changes by taking the games into bed with Ibi. However, the Nintendo is in Sayo's room and is not easily removed, so Ibi still has to go to Sayo's room to play. I asked if he was sad about the situation and he said no. I didn't believe him because I knew he was trying to be a big boy and please me. I told him to let me know if he does feel sad and wants to talk about anything.

Sunday, March 12

Ibi's Entry

I felt very awful through the whole day. My body was achy, and I felt a little depressed. I took my first round of medication, and lay in bed all day. I could not do much with my mind or body. I felt very weak, achy and feverish through the day. I skipped lunch because I had no appetite, but ate dinner.

	Breakfast	Lunch	Dinner
	Hot chocolate and bread	Skipped lunch	Baked turkey with corn and broccoli
Medications	600 mg of Ribavirin		600 mg of Ribavirin
Vitamins	500 mg of C, 400IU of E, Multi-Vitamin		500 mg of C

Kunmi's Entry

Ibi still felt very tired and he slept most of the day. He tried to help clean the house and he did a good job cleaning the first bedroom. I don't know why he even bothered when he should be in bed. I said nothing and let him do what he wanted.

Late that night Ibi mentioned that he has a physical scheduled with his work's health services tomorrow afternoon. This was a surprise to me, but I didn't make an issue of it. He was not sure whether or not to tell them he has Hepatitis B. Since the physical does involve extensive blood tests, they will find out. I suggested that if, during his conversation with the physician, it comes out, he should have him or her contact Dr. Najarian for any information.

Ibi did not feel comfortable at all letting anyone besides me, Sayo and Dr. Najarian know that he has

Hepatitis B. He got very angry with me when I mentioned it to one of my friends. He didn't want others knowing for fear of being isolated, looked down on or pitied. I explained that by talking about it, we may get additional information that may either help us cope better or perhaps, help Dr. Najarian with the treatment. He wouldn't hear of it.

MONDAY, MARCH 13

Ibi's Entry

I felt okay when I woke up, so I took my first round of medication and went to work. I had an appointment for a physical at one p.m. with my work's Health Services. She took blood samples and did a pulmonary check, which I passed. I had to tell the lady that I have Hepatitis B and felt extremely uncomfortable with revealing that information to her.

It would be difficult to go to work with everyone knowing my condition. I wonder if their fear would result in my being asked to stay home for the duration of the treatment. I really need to work to keep my mind occupied during the day. Boredom would make me aware of every side effect of the drug. As it is now, I am really struggling to ignore the fatigue, aches and fevers. What would my manager think about the secrecy? How will everyone now perceive me? Numerous other thoughts raced through my mind as I walked back to the office. I did not ask the physician if she was going to report all the information to my manager or director. I'll wait and see what happens.

As I walked back to the office, I also wondered if there was a corrollation between the effect of the drugs and time I eat. I had a late lunch to test if there will be other reactions than the ones I already have with the medication. I wondered if the drug works better on an empty system.

As soon as I got back in my office, I called Dr. Najarian to let him know what happened with my job's physician. He took the woman's name and said he would handle it. I made an appointment with him for 5:45 p.m. on Wednesday.

	Breakfast	Lunch	Dinner
	Two rolls of bread and hot chocolate	Steak and cheese sub	Baked turkey with corn and broccoli
Medications	600 mg of Ribavirin		.2cc Interferon, 600 mg of Ribavirin, 1ml white count booster hormone
Vitamins	500 mg of C, 400IU of E, Multi-Vitamin		500 mg of C

Kunmi's Entry

Ibi woke up tired as usual. We discussed what he should say to the doctor. I called him late in the afternoon to see how the physical went and he did not return my call. At night, he said he had to tell the woman he had Hepatitis B. She wanted more details and he referred her to Dr. Najarian. I was a bit concerned about whether or not she will mention it to his manager.

We talked about possible consequences and how he should react to them. *Consequence:* They ask him to stay home for fear of their being infected. *Reaction:* He would educate them about Hepatitis and how it is contracted to reassure them that they are in no danger. If they still insist, he would stay home. We would then be on a one-person income because his job does not have short-term disability benefit. It would be financially tight. *Consequence:* Why the secrecy? *Reaction:* He'll explain that he is a private person, and since he did not see them being infected by him, there was no need to tell them.

TUESDAY, MARCH 14

Ibi's Entry

I woke up feeling achy and a little feverish, but I went to work anyway. When I took my first round of medication, I realized that I didn't have much of an appetite for food, but I forced myself to eat anyway.

My work's doctor called me about the results of my blood test and physical. She told me my white count was very low. I told her to fax a copy of the results to Dr. Najarian. She also told me that her husband is a Hepatologist and recommended I seek treatment from him.

I called my doctor later for blood test results. He said that I should increase the hormone to three times a week. He said if my white blood count stays low, we might have to stop the treatment. I couldn't believe what he said and asked him to repeat it. I was in major depression. This would mean that I would have to live with Hepatitis for the rest of my life. It may or may not lead to other health problems in the future. I hung up the phone, sat at my desk quietly doing nothing for the rest of the afternoon. I felt very tired from that time on.

I picked Sayo up, gave him dinner and sent him upstairs to play with our tenant's two children. I lay in bed after I took my second round of medication and slept. Our tenant sent Sayo down around eight p.m and he went to bed immediately. I went back to sleep and woke up around 11:30 p.m. and ironed my clothes.

	Breakfast	Lunch	Dinner
	Quaker Oats	Broiled salmon and vegetables	Chinese food
Medications	600 mg of Ribavirin		600 mg of Ribavirin
Vitamins	500 mg of C, 400IU of E, Multi-Vitamin		500 mg of C

Kunmi's Entry

Ibi developed a fever overnight and still had it in the morning, yet he went to work. I got home very late from school. He was asleep, but woke up as soon as I entered the room. I thought someone had died from the look on his face and regretted coming home so late, but I didn't have a choice, I had a group meeting with my classmates. I asked if everything and everyone was okay. I knew Sayo was fine because I had checked on him when I walked in.

Ibi sat up on the bed and told me that he may be stopping the treatment. I was shocked, motionless and had to sit down. I knew that he must be very depressed about the news because of the look on his face. I was not going to accept the possibility. I have been fasting faithfully for the pasting sixteen days and refused to believe that it was in vain. I reassured him and told him to have faith. He wished he could fast also this lent but is unable to due to his treatment, but he does pray. I suggested that we both need to pray more and that everything will be fine. I gave him a hug and stroked his head until he fell asleep. I am extremely frustrated with this treatment because nothing seems to be working.

WEDNESDAY, MARCH 15

Ibi's Entry

I woke up feeling okay but a little tired. I took my first round of medication before I went to work.

I left work for my appointment with my doctor. He discussed the blood results from my work's doctor with me in detail. The results were similar to the ones he had previously done.

I suggested to Dr. Najarian that I change the times I administer the hormone. I felt that since we have not seen the desired result, it wouldn't hurt to try the medications my way. I told him that I think the Interferon works well when I use it with the hormone. I suggested that we try using the hormone and Interferon on the same day, at the same time. Without telling my doctor, I tried the hormone on Monday evening to see how it worked with the other medications. I felt very sick from the side effects of the Interferon, which was supposed to make me feverish, and it did. Since I felt this way, I knew the Interferon was working.

I came home and took the second round of my medication and went to bed right away. I got a good night's sleep.

	Breakfast	Lunch	Dinner
	Hot chocolate	Chinese lobster sauce and white rice	Baked potato with turkey stew
Medications	600 mg of Ribavirin		600 mg of Ribavirin
Vitamins	500 mg of C, 400IU of E, Multi-Vitamin		500 mg of C

Kunmi's Entry

Ibi looked tired. He was asleep when Sayo and I got home at nine p.m. He didn't even wake up. He sort of turned around and went back to sleep.

Thursday, March 16

Ibi's Entry

I woke up feeling okay. I had breakfast and forgot to take my medication. I was busy at work but managed to find time for lunch. I lost track of time and did not realize what time it was. I rushed to Sayo's school to pick him up. I forgot to call my doctor today. I wanted to catch him before he left his office. I called him when I got home.

It seems that I am more forgetful since the treatment started. Kunmi reminds me a good amount of the time to make an entry into my journal. Sometimes, I forget things that happen earlier in the day

I talked to my doctor and he told me the results of my blood tests looked very promising. He told me my white blood count was very high and that my platelets were low. He said the enzymes were high, and it was expected that the virus would most likely be destroyed. He said no one had ever researched using Interferon or Ribavirin with the white blood hormone. He said he might write it up as a study and that so far, the treatment looked very promising. He felt very positive about my cure. I felt positive too.

I took my first round of medication and the hormone injection around six p.m. I hope to take the Interferon and the second round of medication before I sleep tonight. I was feeling stronger than yesterday.

	Breakfast	Lunch	Dinner
	Hot chocolate	Rice with turkey stew, an apple	Two cans of clam chowder and bread
Medications	600 mg of Ribavirin		600 mg of Ribavirin
Vitamins	500 mg of C, 400IU of E, Multi-Vitamin		500 mg of C

Kunmi's Entry

Ibi said that he felt sicker with the hormone. Dr. Najarian called and said that it looked as though the medicine was working. I was so excited. Ibi is his grouchy old self. He didn't seem excited about the news. I thought maybe he didn't hear the news and repeated it twice and he nodded, and showed no excitement.

FRIDAY, MARCH 17

Ibi's Entry

I woke up today wishing the day was almost over. I did not feel like going to work but went anyway. I had my first round of medication and breakfast before I left. I had a busy day at work, but I felt motivated because of the new positive hopes from my doctor. I finished work and was feeling tired. I picked Sayo up at school, came home and gave him dinner.

I took my second round of medication and went to bed. I was relieved to know that there was not going to be any work tomorrow.

	Breakfast	Lunch	Dinner
	Hot chocolate	Fried chicken, corn and biscuit	Lasagna
Medications	600 mg of Ribavirin		600 mg of Ribavirin
Vitamins	500 mg of C, 400IU of E, Multi-Vitamin		500 mg of C

Kunmi's Entry

Ibi seemed tired. He didn't feel like going to work, but he went because his manager was out on vacation. He was in bed when I got home. He still didn't seem excited about the treatment. I guess it is a defense mechanism in that he didn't want to get his hopes up, should there not be a cure. He said it was premature for celebration.

Saturday, March 18

Ibi's Entry

I woke up well rested and took my first round of medication. I did some cleaning around the house, but all of a sudden, I felt very tired. I had to go back to bed. I was running a fever, but I went to work for about an hour and a half anyway. I took my hormone and Interferon injections two hours later. I lay in bed and studied all night. I took my second round of medication.

	Breakfast	Lunch	Dinner
	Hot chocolate and Quaker Oats	Nigerian Cuisine - Amala and fresh fish peppered stew	Rice and stew
Medications	600 mg of Ribavirin		.2cc Interferon, 600 mg of Ribavirin, 1ml white count booster hormone
Vitamins	500 mg of C, 400IU of E, Multi-Vitamin		500 mg of C

Kunmi's Entry

Ibi dreaded taking his medicine. I was about to enter the bedroom and noticed him picking up the syringe and putting it down twice and I could understand why. I credit him for sticking with it this long. It is difficult to undergo this treatment. I hid behind the door for about five minutes and watched him stare at the syringes. He was startled as I entered the room. I asked if I could be of help and he said no. Within a few seconds, he had injected both.

Later that night, I was cranky as ever. I am sick of school, work and Ibi's illness. I went out and drove around for a while, but it didn't help.

SUNDAY, MARCH 19

Ibi's Entry

I woke up feeling achy and feverish. I took my first round of medication and laid back in bed. Later, we all went to the movies. It was very interesting. We drove to Revere, Massachusetts for dinner. I came home and ironed my clothes for work. I did some studying and took my second round of medication before I went to bed.

	Breakfast	Lunch	Dinner
	Chicken stew with egg and bread	Baked pork chops with potatoes and vegetables	Roast beef sandwich, fries and soda
Medications	600 mg of Ribavirin		600 mg of Ribavirin
Vitamins	500 mg of C, 400IU of E, Multi-Vitamin		500 mg of C

Kunmi's Entry

I felt better about life and Ibi seems okay. His fever, aches and pain have become part of our everyday life and it's not considered an illness. He manages to go to work and do chores in the house.

Later that day Ibi was feeling very good, but confessed dreading the injection. I asked if he wanted me to inject him. After all, I was a nursing student for a year. He said no. This was an interesting side of him I had not seen. He was actually afraid of something. I looked at him as a child who had so many fears and uncertainty inside and was afraid to let them show. I was glad that he said something about this because it showed he was comfortable with me and knew I would be sympathetic. He waited a few hours longer than usual to inject himself. This is the third or so time he had taking his medications late. I wonder if there are any repercussions.

MONDAY, MARCH 20

Ibi's Entry

I woke up feeling good and went to work. I had my first round of medication before I left. I was a little confused about what to do with the database at work. I was to build a database to keep track of the radiation materials. I couldn't decide which database program and structure would be best suited to our needs.

Not quite an hour after I got to work, Kunmi called me about her car's brake pads falling out. I had to give her my car. She dropped her car at a nearby mechanic to be fixed. I will pick it up when I close at five. The car did not get fixed today. She had to rush to pick me at work and also make her class. I called Roberta to pick Sayo up for me, and I picked him up from her house later. I tried to study, but I was too tired.

I tried another experiment of my own. I was curious to see how my body would react when the hormone and Interferon are taken the same day, but at different times. I took the hormone two hours before I took the Interferon injection. I took the remaining medication an hour after the Interferon and went to sleep.

	Breakfast	Lunch	Dinner
	Quaker Oats and hot chocolate	Fish and chips	Three hot dogs with bread
Medications	600 mg of Ribavirin		.2cc Interferon, 600 mg of Ribavirin, 1ml white count booster hormone
Vitamins	500 mg of C, 400IU of E, Multi-Vitamin		500 mg of C

Kunmi's Entry

Ibi missed his father's call in the morning. I was pleased that he called to check on Ibi's health.

I heard something heavy fall below my foot as I drove off after leaving Sayo at school. I immediately lost control of my brakes. I was so grateful that I was not on the highway, where it would have caused a fatal accident. I was still in Cambridge, so I turned around, headed to an automotive shop in Boston near Ibi. I took his car to work.

Later in the evening, Ibi seemed in good spirits. He called his sister-in-law in New York, Sonia, to tell her about his health and that her daughter, Toks, his niece, was to be included in our wedding.

Tuesday, March 21

Ibi's Entry

To my surprise, I am more clear headed than I had been these past two to three weeks. This made me feel positive about the treatment. I also felt a little stronger than I usually feel. I took my first round of medication and went to work.

There was a lot to do as soon as I got to work. I had a busy day as usual. I felt really tired after lunch. I met my director, and he told me if I needed some time off or would like to be excused from certain duties, I should let him or my manager know. Apparently, the health services' doctor did not tell them I have Hepatitis, but that I have a condition that may limit my performance. That felt good. My director went on to say that I was to receive a raise and that in July he would reevaluate my level of responsibility for an upgrade.

I called my doctor for my antigen test. He told me the virus was still present, but I should not worry about it. He said we were on the right track.

I picked up the car from the mechanic and Sayo at

school and came home. I felt tired at the end of the day. I got home and fed Sayo some rice. I ate the leftover oats in the refrigerator. I went to bed and slept till eight p.m. before I took my second round of medication. My doctor called about 7:45 p.m. to inform me about the other e-Antigen test that he was expecting. He told me this test was negative, and he thinks we will be able to cure the disease. He sounded very excited on the phone. I was still very sleepy so I did not sound very excited. But after I hung up the phone, reality set in and I yelled for joy. I could feel the happiness inside me. I could not wait to see Kunmi. I couldn't wait for her to come home so I could tell her.

	Breakfast	Lunch	Dinner
	Banana bread, hot chocolate	Whopper, fries and large soda	Quaker Oats
Medications	600 mg of Ribavirin		600 mg of Ribavirin
Vitamins	500 mg of C, 400IU of E, Multi-Vitamin		500 mg of C

Kunmi's Entry

Ibi met me at the door and told me that the Hepatitis Antigen is negative, gone. The medicine is working. I was so excited but he acted calm and collected. He said Dr. Najarian called and also sounded excited. He suggested buying stock in ICN to help us out financially, the treatment has been expensive because we had to pay cash for all the Ribavirin medication. We also paid for the trip to Mexico.

We talked about writing a book to document the treatment. No one should have to go through this treatment without a resource.

Ibi complained about aches on both arms at night. This happened earlier in the treatment and am not sure why it had returned now. I had Ibi call Dr. Najarian. He said to see how Ibi felt in the morning and to give him a call if there is no change. Ibi took two Tylenol later that night and fell asleep.

WEDNESDAY, MARCH 22

Ibi's Entry

I woke up feeling stronger than yesterday. There was no pain in my arms. I was also feeling very excited about the news Dr. Najarian gave me about the e-antigen test being negative. I had breakfast and took my first round of medication. I went to work and was busy as usual. My manager told me that we should wrap up the laser eye protection project, which was to determine which eye guard was best in protecting the eyes of those exposed to laser beams during their experiments. There are new projects coming in. Things are going well with the database entries by the work-study student.

I went to see my doctor at around 5:20 p.m. and he took my blood samples. He warned me that I should look out for bleeding that does not clot. He said my platelets were a little bit lower than normal. He also explained that the stage we were at on my treatment is for my enzymes to clear up; it will then stabilize, which shows that the medication is working. After it clears up, the level will drop. He went through my blood results with me. Everything looked good and promising.

I stopped by the drug store to pick up a box of the hormones. I came home, had dinner and studied UNIX.

	Breakfast	Lunch	Dinner
	Quaker Oats	Whopper, fries and soda	Nigerian Cuisine - Jollof rice, turkey and corn
Medications	600 mg of Ribavirin		600 mg of Ribavirin
Vitamins	500 mg of C, 400IU of E, Multi-Vitamin		500 mg of C

Kunmi's Entry

Ibi looked good, calm and in high spirits. He showed me papers about the e-antigen being negative. It says none was detected. For the first time in our three-year relationship, he seemed a little excited about something. Ibi went to sleep between 7:30 p.m. and eight. He was very tired, and so was I.

THURSDAY, MARCH 23

Ibi's Entry

I woke up feeling good with no pains or aches. I had breakfast and took my first round of medication with juice. I packed some lunch for work. I ate my lunch around one p.m. I kept myself very busy at work, and I tried to concentrate on my responsibilities so that I was occupied throughout the whole day. I picked Sayo up at school, and we came home. I took my second round of medications with juice. I also took my hormone injection.

	Breakfast	Lunch	Dinner
	Quaker Oats, cranberry juice	Rice and stew	Whopper, fries and soda, cranberry juice
Medications	600 mg of Ribavirin		600 mg of Ribavirin, 1ml white count booster hormone
Vitamins	500 mg of C, 400IU of E, Multi-Vitamin		500 mg of C

Kunmi's Entry

I went to efficacy training and did not get to eat breakfast. It was a good program. The training focused on how to understand one's situation and to positively move forward. There was the concept of getting out of a box and recognizing all the forces that work against one to keep that person in the box. The box represents any given situation(s). For me it was dealing and coping with Ibi's illness, as well as handling issues with school and work. The program was taught using various exerises and games. It also taught how to set up support systems for oneself. This class was good therapy for me considering all that is happening with Ibi.

Ibi was already in bed when I got home, tired. I was tired too, so I went to bed.

FRIDAY, MARCH 24

Ibi's Entry

I woke up feeling stressed and exhausted, so I took the day off from work. Kunmi's sister-in-law Kemi and brother M.T. had dropped their dog off for me to babysit for the weekend so I stayed home and played with him. I love dogs and it would have been great to have one in the house throughout the treatment. I could walk him which is great for thinking, play fetch and just have fun. I really miss not having a dog.

I took my first round of medication. I slept for a few hours later and felt really rested. After reading about twenty pages of the UNIX administration guide, I was tired again. Hearing that Michael Jordan will play on TV raised my spirits. I took the dog for a walk after watching the game. During the walk, I thought back on the treatment and my feelings. I realized that I have been and am easily irritated.

I took my second round of medication after this. I went to bed very late.

	Breakfast	Lunch	Dinner
	Rice and stew, hot chocolate	Two hot dogs	Chicken and vegetables
Medications	600 mg of Ribavirin		600 mg of Ribavirin
Vitamins	500 mg of C, 400IU of E, Multi-Vitamin		500 mg of C

Kunmi's Entry

Ibi seemed in good spirits and not tired. He had blood work done.

I had another day of efficacy. We did group exercises in which we were presented several problems and had to resolve them. Even though these were games, I learned a great deal about myself. I don't deal with failure too well. I always play to win. If Ibi does not get cured, I would probably be more miserable than him because I wouldn't accept that the medications just did not do what they were supposed to do.

At the end of today's efficacy program, we were instructed to get into a group of three, called our success team, and make a list of short-term goals to work on. The efficacy class meets for another two days in April. We were to help each other achieve these goals by the next time we meet. Ways to cope better with Ibi's withdrawal and forgetfulness were on my list. I listed possible resources to tap into next to each goal.

Saturday, March 25

Ibi's Entry

I woke up feeling good. I read some computer update newsletters. Later I let the dog out to go to the bathroom. When we came back in, I had breakfast and my first round of medication. I had breakfast and gave the dog his food. He didn't like his food, so I gave him some of mine.

It was a calm day. I went to the store for a little while, came back and took my hormone injection. Three hours later, I took the Interferon injection. Kunmi and I had dinner. We went shopping for Sayo's birthday party in the evening.

	Breakfast	Lunch	Dinner
	Oat bran cereal	Two cheeseburgers	Hot chocolate and Quaker Oats
Medications	600 mg of Ribavirin		.2cc Interferon, 600 mg of Ribavirin, 1ml white count booster hormone
Vitamins	500 mg of C, 400IU of E, Multi-Vitamin		500 mg of C

Kunmi's Entry

Ibi bought two birthday cards for Sayo. We bought candy and birthday take-away goodies bags. I was confused about what to get and Ibi took over. He asked how many children were coming and I told him. Since he and Sayo spent more time together he knew which theme was best and picked all that was needed using that theme. I basically followed him around in the store as he made his selection. Occassionally, he glanced at me, shook his head and smiled.

Then we went to the grocery store. I was very irritated, everything annoyed me. Ibi made us start at the first aisle. He picked the items he thought we needed and asked about the ones he wasn't sure about.

I was overwhelmed with the thoughts of finishing school, planning a wedding, taking care of a sick fiancé, a son, a house and dealing with the pressures of work.

I felt better after I ate. Ibi was accommodating; he's so sweet and wonderful. I think in his own way he felt really sorry for me. It is difficult to discern what he is feeling and thinking. He always says I am not satisfied unless I have problems to deal with, and when the problems find me, I complain. He did not say that today, but I know he is thinking it. No matter how much I nagged and complained, he was quiet or tried to say something positive. He even tried a joke or two. I was in no mood to laugh.

When we got home, I packed Sayo's party favors. Ibi gave me a long bear hug, then we slept.

SUNDAY, MARCH 26

Ibi's Entry

I woke up feeling very sore in the muscles, and I also felt very tired than usual. It may be due to all the work I did yesterday. We had to do all that we did yesterday for today to be successful and Kunmi seems to be having a crisis. I handled the situation the best I knew how.

After I had breakfast, I went right back to bed. I slept for two hours then got ready for Sayo's birthday party. It was in Peabody, which was a thirty-minute drive. We all had fun playing games. I played all the games. Hours went by and I felt no aches or pain. I had so much fun, I felt better going into the next day.

	Breakfast	Lunch	Dinner
	Egg sandwich	Skipped lunch	Pizza, salad, breadsticks and soda
Medications	600 mg of Ribavirin		600 mg of Ribavirin
Vitamins	500 mg of C, 400IU of E, Multi-Vitamin		500 mg of C

Kunmi's Entry

We went to an indoor family playground for Sayo's birthday party. All our family and friends showed up. We ate pizza, salad and drank to our heart's content. All the kids and adults played games, and I had a great time with the alligator that sticks out its head and if you hit it quickly enough, you get a certain amount of points. Ibi and the boys were playing ping-pong, basketball and video games. If adults were allowed on the children's rides, Ibi would be first in line. He was having more fun than the children. I wondered if he remembered to take his medication this morning because there were no signs of fatigue, fever, aches or pains. We all had a great time. I hope we can all do it together again next year, God willing.

At bedtime, I saw Ibi taking his medication and asked if he took them in the morning and he said he did. I sat on the bed, facing Ibi and thanked him for being there and supportive. Despite his treatment, he was physically able to handle all the shopping yesterday and put all the groceries away when we got home. This morning, he made sure that all that we needed to take to the indoor playground was put in the car. He looked at me, smiled and said that is what relationships were for. We hugged, kissed and went to bed.

MONDAY, MARCH 27

Ibi's Entry

I woke up feeling okay. I had a seminar all this week and I was loaded with a lot of information. I was okay through the day.

I took my medications with the hormone injection when I got home and Interferon two hours later. I did more reading and went to bed.

	Breakfast	Lunch	Dinner
	Potato and stew	Tuna sandwich	Sloppy Joe
Medications	600 mg of Ribavirin		.2cc Interferon, 600 mg of Ribavirin, 1ml white count booster hormone
Vitamins	500 mg of C, 400IU of E, Multi-Vitamin		500 mg of C

Kunmi's Entry

I got a call from my mentor about feedback from a person with whom I took the efficacy class. It was about a comment I supposedly made about my mentor leaving the Diversity Advisory Group at work. This person in the efficacy program had misinterpreted what I said about my mentor retiring from the committee, had told her, and she was upset. I was disturbed. I came home and told Ibi and he was not supportive. "I told you so", he said. I was angry at the efficacy classmate. I was more angry at Ibi. I expected him to be supportive; he usually is. It must be the medication. One minute, Ibi is compassionate and delicate in pointing out my mistakes, the next minute, he is cold and uncaring. I slept in Sayo's room.

TUESDAY, MARCH 28

Ibi's Entry

I did not feel good this morning. I felt sour and feverish, but I could not stay home because I didn't want to miss out on the seminar. I was not sure when it would be possible to go again, so I took my morning medication and left home.

I felt tired in the morning, but with time, I started feeling better. I am not sure why this morning is different from other mornings. I have not changed my medication, the dose or time taken. I also don't understand why I feel okay one minute and feel exhausted the next. I came home exhausted. I took my second round of medication and went to bed for a while. I woke up later and did some reading.

	Breakfast	Lunch	Dinner
	Quaker Oats	Sausage, onion and pepper sub	Sloppy Joe
Medications	600 mg of Ribavirin		600 mg of Ribavirin
Vitamins	500 mg of C, 400IU of E, Multi-Vitamin		500 mg of C

Kunmi's Entry

No entry.

WEDNESDAY, MARCH 29

Ibi's Entry

I woke up feeling really sleepy and tired. I took my morning medication with breakfast and went to work. I spent a busy day trying to assimilate a lot of information. I made it through the day and came home. I took my second round of medication, lay down in bed for a while and wrote my memo. I felt very depressed yesterday and also some part of today. I tried to face reality by making myself aware of what was going on around me. I also tried to figure out what was wrong and what was causing me to feel this way.

Depression is a very hard thing to fight. You need to have a very strong mind that will maintain its focus and direction even in the time of confusion. The way I deal with depression is by keeping myself occupied. I watch a lot of television and will change the channel the minute I don't find it interesting. I also try to keep myself very busy by getting involved with the UNIX program, which is very challenging to learn.

It helps to have someone who forces you to be busy. For me it was Sayo. Whether I wanted to or not, I played Nintendo. Kunmi picks up where Sayo leaves off.

	Breakfast	Lunch	Dinner
	Hot chocolate and a slice of bread	Middle Eastern food - Filafia	Rice and stew
Medications	600 mg of Ribavirin		600 mg of Ribavirin
Vitamins	500 mg of C, 400IU of E, Multi-Vitamin		500 mg of C

Kunmi's Entry

I was still very upset about Ibi not being supportive when I told him about the situation between me, my mentor and the efficacy classmate. He implied I deserved it and used a totally unrelated past situation, to justify his point. I became angry and said things I didn't mean.

Some woman came to look at the tenant's damaged tiles and gave an estimate as to the repair cost. It was too expensive. As soon as she left, we resumed our conversation and we both ended up being angry. We both stopped listening to each other. It occurred to me that his behavior might be the result of the medication. I was not going to excuse it even if that's a factor.

THURSDAY, MARCH 30

Ibi's Entry

I woke up still feeling sleepy. I took my shower and got ready to attend the seminar I've been going to all this week. I took my morning medication and left home. I keep praying that this treatment will be successful. I would like to live a normal and healthy life. I am tired of all these medications. I am tired of the aches, pains and fevers. I am tired of the exhaustion and constant change of moods. Sometimes, I barely make it through a work day and when I do, I wonder how I managed.

I stopped by Sayo's school to pick him up and fed him when I got home. I took my hormone injection and about an hour and a half later, I took the Interferon injection.

Kunmi came home early, and we spent time together. I realized that every time I am running a temperature and Kunmi caresses me all over, my temperature falls back to normal. I also took my second round of medication before I went to bed.

	Breakfast	Lunch	Dinner
	Pancakes and sausage	Turkey and roast beef sandwiches	Turkey noodle soup
Medications	600 mg of Ribavirin		.2cc Interferon, 600 mg of Ribavirin, 1ml white count booster hormone
Vitamins	500 mg of C, 400IU of E, Multi-Vitamin		500 mg of C

Kunmi's Entry

It was a hectic day. Ibi seemed fine. There was no significant change to record.

FRIDAY, MARCH 31

Ibi's Entry

I woke up feeling very sour and feverish. I went to my seminar and took my morning medication. I had a headache but I refused to take any other medication. I felt medicated enough. This lasted all day till I got home.

I laid in bed for some time and watched TV to unwind for the day. I found out that when I unwind I can sleep better at night. I did some studying. I took my second round of medication and went to bed.

	Breakfast	Lunch	Dinner
	Quaker Oats	Tuna, crabmeat, turkey sandwiches	Nigerian Cuisine - Eba and Egusi stew with gizzard, kidney & beef tripe
Medications	600 mg of Ribavirin		600 mg of Ribavirin
Vitamins	500 mg of C 400IU of E Multi-Vitamin		500 mg of C

Kunmi's Entry

I got home at nine p.m. and Ibi was upset because I did not have class nor did I tell him I was not coming home directly. This was the first time he ever complained about me being late. It's kind of nice to know that he missed me. Overall he seems fine.

Chapter Seven

It is the mind that makes

Saturday, April 1

Ibi's Entry

I woke up feeling a little bit tired. I did some house cleaning and waited for the tile man to fix the tenants' bathroom. Other contractors showed up to work on other repairs in the tenants' apartment.

I laid down later, and I took my medication in the afternoon. We also went to a major hardware store to buy wall panels. We came back and tried to install the panels in the tenant's apartment, but I could not do it because my whole body ached. I took my hormone shot before we started the paneling work.

I then took my Interferon shot after I quit working. I was feeling very depressed. It might have to do with the unplanned spending for the tenant's repairs. I tried to hang in there. We did not go to sleep early because we did some home budgeting.

	Breakfast	Lunch	Dinner
	Hot chocolate and bread	Leftovers in refrigerator	Nigerian Cuisine - Rice, beans and fried plantains
Medications	600 mg of Ribavirin		Forgot to take Ribavirin
Vitamins	500 mg of C, 400IU of E, Multi-Vitamin		500 mg of C

Kunmi's Entry

The tile man fixed the tenant's tiles for one hundred and fifty dollars. We went to hardware store for other supplies. Ibi and I had a disagreement about how to put the wall covering up. He got angry and left. I attempted to do it by myself, with minimal success, so I quit too. He went in and wrote checks for the monthly bills. I think he forgot to take his Ribavirin before going to bed.

SUNDAY, APRIL 2

Ibi's Entry

I woke up feeling kind of sore. I stayed in bed longer to get more rest. We did some work around the house and also waited on contractors to look at the tenants' apartment. I had to make up for my missed second round of medication last night. I noticed that my tiredness is beginning to extend to my mind. I am becoming more forgetful. At the end of the day I was back at equilibrium on my medication.

We also went grocery shopping. We put the groceries away, had dinner, and went to bed. We also spent some time paying more bills. I woke up at about three a.m. and could not go back to sleep.

	Breakfast	Lunch	Dinner
	Skipped breakfast	Noodles and corn	Nigerian Cuisine - Fried plantains and stew
Medications	600 mg of Ribavirin		600 mg of Ribavirin
Vitamins	500 mg of C, 400IU of E, Multi-Vitamin		500 mg of C

Kunmi's Entry

People came to give us estimates for the carpentry work we need done. It was a good day. We didn't fight today about the paneling work that we didn't do yesterday. We both agreed to hire someone to put them up.

Ibi seems to be in a better mood. He asked if he took his medicine last night and I told him he took his shots, but not the Ribavirin. It bothered me that Ibi forgot to take his Ribavirin. It seemed that he had mastered the routine of taking his medications. I was not surprised because I have noticed he forgets other things, for example, being home at a designated time to watch Sayo so that I can go to school.

To apply the efficacy's concept of getting out of a box, I decided remind him twice a day to make sure he was taking the medications at the correct times.

MONDAY, APRIL 3

Ibi's Entry

I woke up still feeling sleepy, but I went to work anyway. I took my morning medication with breakfast. I could not finish the hot dog; I had little appetite. I was busy as usual at work. I had lunch and this food easily filled me up.

At the end of the day, I went to pick Sayo up at school. I fed him rice and I took my hormone injection while he was eating. About three hours later, I took the Interferon injection. I did some work on the computer and also did some studying on the UNIX operating system. I went to bed very late, about midnight.

	Breakfast	Lunch	Dinner
	Hot chocolate and hot dog	Grapes, yogurt, banana and turkey sandwich	Chinese rice, beef with brocolli and boneless spareribs
Medications	600 mg of Ribavirin		.2cc Interferon, 600 mg of Ribavirin, 1ml white count booster hormone
Vitamins	500 mg of C, 400IU of E, Multi-Vitamin		500 mg of C

Kunmi's Entry

No entry.

TUESDAY, APRIL 4

Ibi's Entry

I found it very hard to get out of bed this morning. The good thing is that I do not feel as sore and feverish as I used to feel after taking the hormone and Interferon injection. I managed to get out of bed. I took my first round of medication. I later left work to pick up Sayo, fed him and took my second round of medication.

	Breakfast	Lunch	Dinner
	Grapefruit, egg sandwich, yogurt and a banana	Middle Eastern sandwich - chicken and bean sprouts	Spaghetti and meatballs, milk
Medications	600 mg of Ribavirin		.2cc interferon, 600 mg of Ribavirin, 1ml white count booster hormone
Vitamins	500 mg of C, 400IU of E, Multi-Vitamin		500 mg of C

Kunmi's Entry

I felt really depressed around one p.m. because my department may get laid-off. I felt better and optimistic at about four. I've always trusted the Lord to take care of me, why am I doubting Him now? I am so worried about Ibi's condition and I cannot do anything about it. I wish I could. So far, the treatment seems to be working. For a while, the situation seemed hopeless, but now, it seems like he'll be cured. There's so much I don't have control over.

WEDNESDAY, APRIL 5

Ibi's Entry

I woke up feeling good. I took my morning medication, had breakfast and went to work. I was very busy at work as usual. I went to a buffet for lunch and ate so much and was very full. I also noticed that I had been feeling very depressed about things in general. It has been a real struggle to keep myself focused.

I went to see my doctor, and he took a blood sample to be tested. I had not seen him in two weeks. He told me about a combination study at Massachusetts General Hospital with Floxin and Interferon. He reassured me that he thinks my treatment will be successful. I came home and told Kunmi about it. I took my second round of medication.

	Breakfast	Lunch	Dinner
	Hot chocolate	Chinese rice, egg foo young, boneless spareribs and chicken wings	Turkey soup
Medications	600 mg of Ribavirin		600 mg of Ribavirin
Vitamins	500 mg of C, 400IU of E, Multi-Vitamin		500 mg of C

Kunmi's Entry

WEDNESDAY, APRIL 5 - FRIDAY, APRIL 7

I had an extremely busy weekend and didn't get a chance to make journal entries. I was out of the house by eight a.m. and back home by 10:30 p.m. Poor boys, I am neglecting them.

THURSDAY, APRIL 6

Ibi's Entry

I woke up as usual feeling okay. I don't know what is wrong, but I have not been too happy about things in general. My weight has been steady, I have not gained or lost weight from the beginning of the treatment.

I had a busy day as usual and went back to the Chinese buffet where I ate yesterday. I was looking forward to coming home so that I could get my injection over with. I took the hormone first and two hours later, the Interferon. I also took my second round of medication.

	Breakfast	Lunch	Dinner
	Hot chocolate and a piece of bread	Chinese rice, chow mein, boneless spareribs, chicken	Quaker Oats
Medications	600 mg of Ribavirin		600 mg of Ribavirin
Vitamins	500 mg of C, 400IU of E, Multi-Vitamin		500 mg of C

FRIDAY, APRIL 7

Ibi's Entry

I woke up feeling a little achy and sour, but I went through the day as usual. I also had my first round of medication. When it is Monday, I am always looking forward to Friday. I came home, took my second round of medication, and laid down to get my body rested and also to unwind for the day. I don't remember if I slept or not, but I think I studied for a while before I went to sleep.

	Breakfast	Lunch	Dinner
	Egg sandwich and hot chocolate	Fried chicken	Pizza
Medications	600 mg of Ribavirin		600 mg of Ribavirin
Vitamins	500 mg of C, 400IU of E, Multi-Vitamin		500 mg of C

SATURDAY, APRIL 8

Ibi's Entry

I woke up feeling better but a little depressed. I got out of bed late and took my first round of medication at about noon. I went to a fast food restaurant for lunch. We had a dinner meeting with some friends who were moving out of Massachusetts. I looked forward to the outing because I needed the distraction. We had a good time and ate Indian food. I took my hormone injection before we left home at 6:15 p.m. and took the Interferon around 11:15 p.m. I have not noticed any different body effect from taking my medications late. I took the Interferon before I left because I feel worse if I take all the medications at the same time. I went to sleep as soon as we got home.

	Breakfast	Lunch	Dinner
	Skipped breakfast	Whopper	Indian food - bean soup, curry rice, meat
Medications	600 mg of Ribavirin		.2cc interferon, 600 mg of Ribavirin, 1ml white count booster hormone
Vitamins	500 mg of C, 400IU of E, Multi-Vitamin		500 mg of C

Kunmi's Entry

Ibi had a good time at dinner. It was a chance to have intellectually stimulating conversations with people in the computer industry. It was also a chance to network.

Sayo seems a bit lonesome these days. Since Ibi's treatment began, I tried to keep both of them occupied and entertained. I think Ibi's treatment is getting the better of him and Ibi may not be as much fun to be around as he has been. I decided to have Roberta's son spend the night at our house to keep Sayo company.

SUNDAY, APRIL 9

Ibi's Entry

I woke up feeling okay since I slept till ten a.m. I cleaned the kitchen, did laundry and folded the clothes with Sayo giving me a hand. I took my first round of medication. The day was okay, but I stayed in bed most of the time. I ordered pizza and chicken wings for dinner and I took my second round of medication in the evening. I also ironed my clothes, played around with the computer, and went to bed.

	Breakfast	Lunch	Dinner
	Potato and egg with hot chocolate	Rice, vegetables and turkey stew	Pizza
Medications	600 mg of Ribavirin		600 mg of Ribavirin
Vitamins	500 mg of C, 400IU of E, Multi-Vitamin		500 mg of C

Kunmi's Entry

It was nice to come home to a clean house. Ibi actually put my poor baby, Sayo, to work. I felt sorry for his tiny body folding clothes and vacuuming, but he survived. I peered in his room and he was asleep.

The pizza Ibi ordered tasted awful. I know that I am definitely sick. This is the last thing I need right now.

MONDAY, APRIL 10

Ibi's Entry

I woke up feeling okay and took my first round of medication. I noticed that my vision was blurry and assumed it was because I was not quite awake. I skipped lunch at work because I had a very busy day. Kunmi was feeling sick and did not go to work, but she made us a special dinner. It tasted really good, and we enjoyed it. As soon as I got home, I took my second round of medication and the hormone injection and laid in bed. I woke up around 10:30 p.m. I took my Interferon injection and went back to sleep.

	Breakfast	Lunch	Dinner
	Hot chocolate with milk	Danish and four pieces of cookies	Fish stew, corn and rice
Medications	600 mg of Ribavirin		.2cc Interferon, 600 mg of Ribavirin, 1ml white count booster hormone
Vitamins	500 mg of C, 400IU of E, Multi-Vitamin		500 mg of C

Kunmi's Entry

Ibi needs to see the eye doctor because he can't see. He said things were blurry this morning on his way driving in to work. He wanted to come home at lunch to check on how I was doing, but Dr. Najarian told him not to drive. Apparently, the medication is causing other bodily functions to fail. Early in the treatment, there was worry of damage to the bone marrow. That did not happen, and it was closely watched for. The loss of sight and permanent liver damage were also effects we were warned about.

I was in no condition to go and get him from work. I suggested he take a taxi home. I was upset to see that he drove home and pointed out to him that that decision to drive was not wise. He simply ignored me, as if he did not hear what I said. He took his medicine, ate dinner and went to bed at seven p.m. He couldn't finish the entry in his journal because of the eye pains and fatigue.

TUESDAY, APRIL 11

Ibi's Entry

I felt okay when I woke up. Even though I could see better today, I stayed home. It was extremely difficulty driving home yesterday. I didn't have any money on me and would have had to drive to a money machine, find a telephone and wait for the taxi to arrive. I estimated it would take an hour to do all this. In would be home in less time. So I drove home very slowly and with blinkers on

I took my first round of medication. I skipped lunch but had some chips. I called my doctor and left a message for him requesting information on my blood test. He told me everything was okay, and that was why he did not call. He told me that the flare in my eyes that caused the blurriness might be over because my enzyme level had dropped to about 110.

The major problem I have with this treatment is that it takes a lot of effort to focus my mind through the day, but I always try to keep myself very busy. Kunmi is still feeling sick and did not go to work.

I had leftovers from last night for dinner. I took my second round of medication later.

	Breakfast	Lunch	Dinner
	Fish stew and bread	Chips	Fish stew, corn and rice
Medications	600 mg of Ribavirin		600 mg of Ribavirin
Vitamins	500 mg of C, 400IU of E, Multi-Vitamin		500 mg of C

Kunmi's Entry

No entry.

WEDNESDAY, APRIL 12

Ibi's Entry

I woke up feeling good, with no side effects. My head felt very clear. I took my first round of medication with hot chocolate and went to work. I was very busy at work all day. I came home very tired and took my second round of medication and went to bed very early.

	Breakfast	Lunch	Dinner
	Oat Bran cereal	Rice, peas and Buddha style vegetarian roll	Chinese food
Medications	600 mg of Ribavirin		600 mg of Ribavirin
Vitamins	500 mg of C, 400IU of E, Multi-Vitamin		500 mg of C

Kunmi's Entry
No entry.

THURSDAY, APRIL 13

Ibi's Entry

I woke up feeling very good and excited today for no reason. Kunmi said she was feeling better, and she will be going to work today. I took my first round of medication, as usual, with hot chocolate. I went to work and the day was not too bad. I made a few modifications to the database design. Kunmi did not go to work, instead surprised me at work with lunch. It tasted really good. I introduced her to the people I work with and one person said she was very pretty. It was a good day.

	Breakfast	Lunch	Dinner
	Raisin bread and jelly	Chicken pasta, bread and soup	Rice and stew
Medications	600 mg of Ribavirin		600 mg of Ribavirin
Vitamins	500 mg of C, 400IU of E, Multi-Vitamin		500 mg of C

Kunmi's Entry

I felt vicious today. Ibi talked so much about the girls at work, I had to go see for myself. There is this one girl who gives him a hard time. Either she likes him and he does not pay her attention, or she dislikes him. I wanted them to know that he has a backbone at home, and if they think they can push him around they have something else coming.

So, off I went to an Italian restaurant for some chicken soup and a dozen fresh hot rolls and butter. Ibi was surprised to see me but was glad to see lunch. I went around meeting everyone and offering them a hot roll and butter. I spent enough time with the troublemaking girl to politely make sure she understood my position. And she did and was equally cordial. Ibi needs as little stress as possible, and I cannot have her giving him trouble. I left assured that my mission was accomplished. Besides, everyone complimented my looks. This was a good day.

FRIDAY, APRIL 14 - MONDAY, APRIL 17

Ibi's Entry

No entries.

Kunmi's Entry

Ibi made no entries for the following days and majority of the rest of the month because he was having a crisis. His aches and pains, fevers had returned along with the blurred vision. He was more irritable than ever, everything annoyed him. His appetite varied. He still kept up with his doctor's visit and medications.

He was experiencing more depression than previously and barely said two words. I wondered how he was doing at work. When I ask how he is in general, he just nods and says fine.

He lost total interest in making entries even though he knew their importance. It seemed that he was fed up with the treatment and did not feel like doing any additional things. Making entries into the journal is additional. One might say that he stopped caring.

I had no entry for Saturday, April 15.

Sunday, April 16

Kunmi's Entry

Today is Easter Sunday. Sayo and I went to church. Ibi was tired and wanted to rest. Church service was great.

Tuesday, April 18

Ibi's Entry

I took the day off to relax by myself. I didn't feel like writing or doing anything, so I just slept and rested.

Kunmi's Entry

Ibi stayed home today because he wasn't feeling well. Lately, he's been more tired, irritated and depressed. He also refused to talk about how he is feeling. He wants to be left alone and keeps to himself. He picked Sayo up for me because I had class tonight. He said he slept most of the day. I took my Finance and Marketing exams. I think I passed.

Wednesday, April 19

Ibi's Entry

I felt very healthy today and went to work. I took my morning medication with some hot chocolate, but I skipped breakfast. I had a cheap Chinese noodle lunch. The day was normal, and nothing really exciting happened. I came home and took my second round of medication. I did some work on the computer till very late at night when Kunmi came home.

	Breakfast	Lunch	Dinner
	Hot chocolate	Chinese noodles	Sloppy Joe
Medications	600 mg of Ribavirin		600 mg of Ribavirin
Vitamins	500 mg of C, 400IU of E, Multi-Vitamin		500 mg of C

Kunmi's Entry

I managed to lose about 30 pounds due to fasting and now I have gained 2 pounds. Ibi is still in his mood. I suggested that Ibi send Sayo upstairs to play with the tenants' children until his bedtime. I asked the tenants how much it would be to compensate them, since Sayo may be coming up for a few hours on the weekdays on a regular basis. I felt that Ibi is stressed and he needs to have one less responsibility, Sayo.

Thursday, April 20

Ibi's Entry

I was feeling very good today. I took my first round of medication when I woke up. I don't have much of an appetite, but I always try to eat before taking the medication.

I came home from work and took my hormone injection and two hours later my Interferon injection. I noticed that I have been feeling very depressed for the last four days. I try to find a way to take control of my mind so I do not wander too far. I really don't like the quietness of the house, I wish someone were here.

	Breakfast	Lunch	Dinner
	Hot chocolate and two slices of bread	Large cheeseburger, fries and soda	Baked chicken with broccoli
Medications	600 mg of Ribavirin		600 mg of Ribavirin
Vitamins	500 mg of C, 400IU of E, Multi-Vitamin		500 mg of C

Kunmi's Entry

I was so relieved and happy that Finance and Marketing is over. I called home to check on Ibi, but the phone was just ringing. He did not pick up and I was wondering where he was, since it was nine p.m. and he is usually home by then. I was really worried that something had happened to Ibi or Sayo and no one could reach me. Sayo was with Roberta.

Unfortunately, I couldn't leave Finance because of my presentation. I got to Roberta's house at 10:30 p.m. and nothing was wrong, at least I knew that Sayo was fine. I rushed home and dropped the soundly sleeping Sayo on his bed with his coat and boots on. I dashed for the bedroom to find Ibi motionless on the bed with his back turned to the door. At first I was scared that with the way he laid, he was dead. I put my hand over his nose, and he was breathing, thank God.

I picked up the phone and called Roberta. I asked her to call me back right away, waited five minutes and there was no ring so I called her back. She said the phone rang and I did not pick up. Now I knew the phone was faulty; it rings outside but not inside.

I undressed Sayo and put on his pajamas. I was so tired and joined Ibi in bed. He was snoring loudly and made it difficult for me to fall asleep, so I watched TV.

Friday, April 21

Ibi's Entry
No entry.

Kunmi's Entry

Today was the last day of the efficacy program and it gave me back the control of our lives. Since the last time, we met, I had worked on being more tolerant of the medicinal effects of Ibi's treatment.

The program helped me put things in their proper perspective. When we began his treatment we basically made a conscious decision to get rid of the virus in his body. We did a lot of research on the disease and asked a lot of questions. I tried to do everything to make sure that he will be cured. I prayed and fasted. I planned balanced meals, though we ended up eating out half of the time. I encouraged him to stay home from work and rest, and he refused. I tried to help him keep a positive outlook even when the blood tests were not favorable. I gave this battle with the virus, the box, my all. If that is not enough, I will not be disappointed, but accept that the cure may not be a possibility at this time.

Saturday, April 22

Ibi's Entry
No entry.

Kunmi's Entry

The handyman did not show up as anticipated, so I put a stop payment on his check. I am sure he'll be calling and I'll ask him what his intentions were as to receive money and not perform the job. I wrote up a contract for him and us to sign. Ibi did not seem too concerned about it. This is the last time I will go along with Ibi's way of doing things. At least with a signed contract, I have a recourse to get my money back.

Ibi insisted that we needed a new car, a 4 X 4. He had been searching for prices on the Internet for the last few days and found a dealer he felt we should visit. So, we went car shopping.

SUNDAY, APRIL 23

Ibi's Entry
No entry.

Kunmi's Entry

Ibi and I went to the hardware store to exchange the garbage disposal we bought. We purchased more gardening materials and tools.

I got home at 8:45 p.m. and Sayo was fast asleep. I asked the usual questions such as, did you take your medication, did you feed Sayo, and found out that Ibi forgot to feed him dinner because they were too busy playing Nintendo. He said they had fun. I was very angry at him for not feeding the boy. He apologized.

He later complained about fatigue and body aches. He went to sleep by 9:30 p.m. I was still very angry at him for not feeding Sayo and was not sympathetic to his aches and pains. I was so overwhelmed and depressed with our situation, the treatment, caring for Sayo and school. I depend on Ibi to take care of Sayo and now it seems that the treatment prevents him from performing this task well. I went to sleep after 11 p.m. depressed, angry and tired.

MONDAY, APRIL 24

Ibi's Entry

No entry.

Kunmi's Entry

No entry.

TUESDAY, APRIL 25

Ibi's Entry

No entry.

Kunmi's Entry

Ibi and I were barely speaking this morning. The last few days have been difficult. His mood swings from one extreme to the other. One minute he is energetic, another he is exhausted. One minute he is happy, another he is depressed. And so on and so forth.

At night, things were back to normal for the moment. He was complaining about pains in the area of his stomach where he injects his shots. I got him a hot water bottle to place over the area overnight.

WEDNESDAY, APRIL 26

Kunmi's Entry

I met with my finance group to rehearse for our class presentation. I had to take Sayo with me since Ibi wasn't speaking to me. He didn't believe I was going to my finance meeting and he wanted me to stay home. This was unlike him. I wonder what's gotten into him. I have been to two or more finance meetings prior to now. I offered to leave the phone number of where I would be and he refused.

It seems Ibi is experiencing mental anxiety and possible paranoia from the medication.

THURSDAY, APRIL 27

Kunmi's Entry

Ibi had an emergency at work and came home at nine p.m. He was very sick through the night. He was restless, feverish and complained about everything. He kept me up all night moaning and groaning, and I tried to be sympathetic even though he had been a very difficult person these last two weeks.

FRIDAY, APRIL 28

Kunmi's Entry

Ibi stayed home to rest today. Earlier in the morning and afternoon when I called to see how he was doing, he said he had shortness of breath. I found him in bed very ill and feverish. He told me he has to go to work tomorrow to catch up with his responsibilities, and I told him that he would go over my dead body. He said that it could be arranged, my dead body, that is.

He picked Sayo up from school despite the fact that he was sick. He ordered pizza for Sayo. Sayo seems to be in seventh heaven with all the pizzas, Thai and Chinese food feasts that he has eaten for the past few months. He seems a bit withdrawn and quiet, though. I asked if there was anything wrong and he said no. He then rambled on about some toy that he wants, and of course I said no.

Chapter Eight

This is the day the Lord has made
let us rejoice and be glad in it.

Tuesday, May 9

Ibi's Entry

I have been feeling extremely depressed since the day I stopped writing this memo. I didn't feel like committing my wild thoughts to paper. I was shocked sometimes at the thoughts that crossed my mind. They were severe thoughts of depression and anxiety.

I have been responding well to the treatment. I don't exercise anymore because my body can't take the strain at this point. I am looking forward to getting the treatment over with. It has restricted my advancement in a lot of ways. I am physically and mentally limited. For me to pursue a career as a UNIX administrator, I have to be able to do more studying and spend a lot of time on the computer practicing. I have not been able to do this. I can't strain myself for anything anymore.

	Breakfast	Lunch	Dinner
	Quaker Oats	Turkey sub	Rice and stew
Medications	600 mg of Ribavirin		600 mg of Ribavirin
Vitamins	500 mg of C, 400IU of E, Multi-Vitamin		500 mg of C

Kunmi's Entry

I am very concerned about Ibi these days. He looks so tired, removed, and depressed. He is extremely quiet. I find myself waking up in the middle of the night to make sure that he is still breathing. I monitor and nag him about his medicine and food intake. The nagging seems to really annoy him, and he gets quite cranky. I stopped asking him if he made entries in his journal because it is obvious to me that he does not want to.

I am grateful for the fact that he at least eats and says a few words. I know something is really wrong.

I finally asked him if he was depressed and thinking of killing himself. I was so afraid of the answer that I immediately told him that he can't kill himself because I can't afford to pay the mortgage alone. I then made a joke about my killing him even though he would already be dead. He called me a liar, and smiled. I was glad to see that lost smile. I felt bad because I had neglected him because of school, and he had been so accommodating. I suggested we do something special Memorial Day weekend and he agreed.

Part of the depression seems to be getting to Sayo,

since the two of them are together a great deal. Sayo, too, is very quiet. This really worries me. I absolutely need to spend more time with both of them. Maybe I should let Sayo go spend the weekend with Roberta or another friend, Cindy. This will give him a break. Ibi and I can then go to the movies or something. Then, next week I'll take Sayo to an indoor playground.

TUESDAY, MAY 15 - WEDNESDAY, MAY 17

Ibi's Entry

I woke up feeling okay. I noticed that I have had more energy these days than before. On Saturday, when I took my injection, I felt very restless and feverish, but I tried to sleep it off. I woke up on Sunday, did some cleaning, cut the grass and cleaned the yard. I took all my medication and injections for the day. I am looking forward to seeing my doctor today, for my blood test.

I saw my doctor Tuesday. He took samples of my blood to test for the surface Antigen. He said if it comes out positive, I will have to use Floxin as a third medication. I would use it within two hours of taking my multi-vitamins. I have been taking my medication religiously.

I am starting to really dislike my job at the university. I am starting to feel that I have no control over my work. All they want to give me is trashy work. They have their own goals and I have mine, but we can never meet. I am looking forward to leaving them for a job I will love.

Kunmi's Entry

No entry.

THURSDAY, MAY 18

Ibi's Entry

I have been feeling stronger and have been working harder. I am trying to organize my work in the office so that I can spend the time to improve my computer expertise. My doctor called with great news that the surface Antigen was negative from the last blood test. I was very excited.

He asked if I wanted to stop the treatment right away and I said I would rather go the six months to be doubly sure that I am okay. It took about four months to cure all traces of the virus. This is good and I am very excited. Thanks be to God.

Kunmi's Entry

Ibi called me at work with the news and I was so excited. I was jumping for joy all over the office. I felt the ordeal was over. When I got home and ask Ibi how he felt, he just smiled. He then told me he'll continue the treatment for another month. I was instantly depressed..

The treatment ended officially on June 21. There are no journal entries after the above for two reason. First, Ibi was tired of the writing and still had many of the side effects of Interferon. The fevers, aches, pains, loss of appetite and so on. He was glad to give a reason to stop writing.

Second, I kept writing despite the fact that I had final exams to prepare for and a lot of changes to deal with at work. I kept a journal in a file on the computer at work, and I thought I made a backup copy. Unfortunately, when I switched jobs I misplaced the file. My old computer had been reformated by the time I realized the error.

Chapter Nine

We've come this far by faith.

Reflecting on the treatment.

Ibi's Entry

I am very grateful to God for giving me the strength and the faith to believe in him. Without God, I would not have made it through this treatment. Through his power, I had the support that pulled me through the treatment, I couldn't have done it alone.

This treatment reminded me of the importance of moral support. My mom always offered me this. She said that I can pull through anything as long as I have faith. Her coaching over the years became useful when I thought my life would be cut short by this illness. I want to live long enough to achieve my goals and enjoy my old age.

This treatment has really made me reevaluate my life and appreciate things more. One thing I found out about myself was that I was not scared of death. I know that I have to die one day. The disease and treatment suggested that it might come sooner than expected.

In the back of my mind I believed very strongly that I was going to be cured. Now that I am cured, I look forward to spending time with my family more than ever. I've made them first in whatever decision I am making.

I promised myself that I will protect my family for the rest of my life. They were very supportive of me throughout the treatment. I try not to put myself under too much stress and to get a lot of rest every weekend. I now work hard in giving Sayo, the better values of life.

I have more confidence in taking risks and hope to pass that confident to my son. I'll try to prevent him from making the same mistakes I made growing up. I will also try to make him take responsibility for his actions and his behavior. I hope all the children I have can achieve more than I achieve before I die. I now train my son to set goals for himself and try to achieve the goals without me. Sayo is always very happy and excited when he sets goals and achieves them. I am teaching him how to accept disappointments and also move on in life. He does not take disappointments well, like his mother. I have to always tell him that he'll do better the next time around.

My fiancée is very hard working and puts a lot of unnecessary stress on herself. I am working with her on how to cope with stress, which I seem to do very well. When I was very depressed during the treatment, she always gave me moral support and said she believed I would be cured in less than six months. She was right. I believe she really loves me. I promised to make her happy and support her. I also want to be able to give her the things that she desires, if they are within my reach. The treatment brought us closer and we also realized that we have a great relationship. If either of us decides to end the relationship, we both can never be as happy as we are now. I now truly believe that we are meant for each other.

My belief is that this treatment should be accepted as a cure. I know that if anyone goes through with the right discipline, that person will be cured.

One also needs the support of other people for

motivation and determination. There should be the desire to live life to its fullest. One must be disciplined; that means being free of any substance abuse, that is drugs, alcohol and others.

I realize that people or companies may be impacted financially by the release of this medical breakthrough and therefore, attack the contents of this book and treatment. I am living evidence of the good of this treatment. It has given me the opportunity to be cured of Chronic Hepatitis B and a second chance at life. I am very proud of myself for having the courage to be the first to undergo this treatment. I hope to reach out to others that are infected, to help educate the public about the disease and the cure.

It was difficult for me to accept that I was physically limited, and I tried to keep up. I found the journal entries to be great therapy. The entries gave me a venue to let out the depression, anger and anxiety that I felt.

Kunmi's Entry

Thank God. I thank him for giving me the strength to be there and supportive of Ibi's treatment. It could have been worse. My advice for anyone considering undergoing the treatment is to have some sort of support in place, someone you can count on in any kind of emergency. For those people who live alone, try to socialize so that all you do when you get home is sleep. Have regular appointments with a counselor or therapist. But most importantly, believe that there is a higher power or energy that you can count on to see you through the treatment. One will need that faith some time during the treatment, especially the first few weeks.

Looking back at the treatment, I would change some things. I felt that I was not as supportive as I wanted to be. I would liked to have gone to every doctor's appointment with Ibi. I had to balance my needs with his.

I consider myself quite fortunate to have such an easy going person to deal with.

At the time I wrote the first draft of this book, March 1996, I was emotionally, mentally, physically, and psychologically exhausted. I was six months pregnant, work was not going well, and I was angry at family and non-family members for doing things that annoyed me. Ibi and I had discussed separating. I was just fed up with life.

Since I typed in all entries, both mine and Ibi's, I had a chance to visualize his feelings at the time and most of those difficult days made sense. I wished I had read his entries prior to no, but I couldn't break our promise to not read the other's entries until after the treatment. If I had read it, I wouldn't have been so stressed and would have been better equipped to cope.

The doctor recommended that we wait at least six months before we attempted to have a baby. This time period would allow the drugs to be completely out of Ibi's system. I found out that I was pregnant in October 1995 with the baby due in June 1996. It had not been six months yet. There was a lot of anxiety for me about the baby being normal. Will he or she have any birth defects from the drug? I then decided that God's will be done. If the baby will cause any problems in our life, I trusted that God would provide a means to make things alright. Ultrasound showed a perfectly healthy baby during my seventh month of pregnancy. I was relieved.

This book helped me remember, that is relive the ordeal of the treatment. It put my relationship in a perspective that helped me make an objective decision of what direction the rest of our lives would follow. I realized that the relationship was not as bad as I thought it was, and that if we could go through those six months of hell, we can do many things.

Additionally, the book made me realize how much I love Ibi and how much we are a part of each other's lives. Many people tell us that from an outside point of view, we behave like siblings and best friends.

The treatment brought Sayo and Ibi closer and I like that. They exclude me from many activities, which gives me time to attend to myself. They play video games, go to soccer practice and games; Ibi signed himself up as assistant coach.

I strongly recommend keeping a journal if one goes through this treatment or any other treatment. After it is all over and hopefully one is cured, this journal will be the reminder of one's ordeal and one's strength. It takes a lot of courage to make it through this. Good luck, with whatever one decides, and have faith.

I am glad to say that I successfully completed the MBA program on August 4, 1995. Ibi and I were married on September 3, 1995, and we raising my son, Sayo.

We gave birth to a healthy baby girl, Yewande,
on June 22, 1996.

Yewande has received two of the three hepatitis shots required. Ibi retested for hepatitis on September 27th, 1996 and is still virus negative. We are all living free of hepatitis.

Blood Tests Definitions and Results

Selected blood tests from Ibi's medical reports are listed so that readers, especially those in the medical community can follow the progression of the combination treatment. Definitions are given for non-medical people. These definitions are the authors understanding of the medical terms. Please consult a doctor or medical text book for exact definitions.

Hepatitis patients undergoing other types of treatment could compare their blood work to those listed here for similarity. The reference ranges listed is for males in Ibi's age group.

Pages 172-173 gives almost two years of blood work. Please keep in mind that dates with no entries are dates which those tests were not ordered.

Source: SmithKline Beecham Clinical Laboratories reports.

TEST	*Definition*	*Reference Range*	*Units*
GLUCOSE	Sugar level in the blood. Indicator of diabetes.	FAST: 70-115	MG/DL
GGT	An enzyme indicator that monitors the liver.	0-65	U/L
ALT (SGPT)	Used to monitor status the of the liver.	0-48	U/L
CHOLESTEROL TOTAL	Total cholesterol - fat in the blood	LESS THAN 200	MG/DL
LDL AND RISK FACTOR	Comparing HDL to LDL.		
LDL CHOLESTROL	The bad cholestrol - Low Density Lypoprotein.	0-130	MG/DL (CALC)
CHOLESTEROL /HDL RATIO	The good cholestrol - High Density Lypoprotein.	LESS THAN 4.98	
CBC, PLATELET CT & DIFF	Complete Blood Count of the different blood cell types.		
WHITE BLOOD CELL COUNT	Amount of white blood cells in the body.	3.8-10.8	thous/mcL
RED BLOOD CELLS	Amount of red blood cells in the body.	4.40-5.80	mill/mcL
HEMOGLOBIN	The % of red blood cells in the blood. It holds oxygen and transports it to the cells.	13.8-17.2	G/DL
HEMATOCRIT	Indicator of blood volume.	41.0-50.0	%

TEST	Definition	Reference Range	Units
MCV	Indicator of the quality of red blood cells.	80.0-100.0	fL
MCH	Mean Corpuscular Hemoglobin - mathematical measure of Hemoglobin concentration of average red blood cells.	27.0-33.0	PG
MCHC	Mean Corpuscular Hemoglobin Concentration - mathematical measure of concentration of hemoglobin in grams per 100 Milliliters of red blood cells.	32.0-36.0	%
PLATELET COUNT	Amount of clotting factor in the blood. This is what clots the blood.	130-400	T/UL
NEUTROPHILS	Type of white blood cells. Used for fighting infection. Immacuture white blood cells.	40-75	%
ABSOLUTE NEUTROPHILS (POLYS)	Actual number present.	1500-1700	CELLS /MCL
LYMPHOCYTES	The mature white blood cells. Leukemia patients have an abundance.	16-46	%
ABSOLUTE LYMPHOCYTES	Actual number present.	850-4100	CELLS /MCL
ABSOLUTE MONOCYTES	Total count of another type of white blood cell.	200-1100	CELLS /MCL
FERRITIN	Measurement of iron.	18-350	NG/ML
HEPATITIS PANEL II, ACUTE	Determination of the Hepatitis Infection in the body.		
* HEPATITIS B SURFACE ANTIGEN	Indicator of the Hepatitis B virus.	NONE DETECTED	
* HEPATITIS B CORE IGM AB	Indicator of infection, appears earlier than other indicators.	NONE DETECTED	
* HEPATITIS A IGM ANTIBODY	Indicator of the Hepatitis A infection.	NONE DETECTED	
* HEPATITIS C ANTIBODY	Indicator of Hepatitis C virus.	NON REACTIVE	
HELICOBACTER PYLORI AB	Type of bacteria causes stomach ulcer.		
* IGA AB	Indicator of past infection and immunity.	NEGATIVE	
* IGG AB	Indicator of past infection and immunity.	NEGATIVE	

TEST	*Units*	*Prior to treatment* 11/8/94	*Six days before treatment* 1/12/95	*Two weeks* 2/8/95	*Three weeks* 2/15/95
GLUCOSE	MG/DL	112	117 H	105	95
GGT	U/L	128 H	152 H	120 H	112 H
ALT (SGPT)	U/L	58 H	61 H	60 H	58 H
CHOLESTEROL TOTAL	MG/DL	229 H	232 H	168	155
LDL AND RISK FACTOR					
LDL CHOLESTROL	MG/DL (CALC)	147 H	145 H		
CHOLESTEROL /HDL RATIO	LESS THAN 4.98	4.24	4.46		
CBC, PLATELET CT & DIFF					
WHITE BLOOD CELL COUNT	thous/mcL	3.8	3.1 L	2.2 L	2.3 L
RED BLOOD CELLS	mill/mcL	4.44	4.52	3.85 L	3.68 L
* HEMOGLOBIN	G/DL	14.7	14.3	12.3 L	11.8 L
* HEMATOCRIT	%	43.3	43.8	38.0 L	37.5 L
* MCV	fL	97.4	96.8	98.7	101.9 H
* MCH	PG	33.1 H	31.7	32.0	32.0
* MCHC	%	33.9	32.7	32.4	31.4 L
* PLATELET COUNT	T/UL	197	200	187	183
NEUTROPHILS	%	39	39		33
ABSOLUTE NEUTRO -PHILS (POLYS)	CELLS /MCL	1482 L	1209 L		
FERRITIN	NG/ML		614 H		1230 H
HEPATITIS PANEL II, ACUTE					
* HEPATITIS BE ANTIBODY			POSITIVE		
* HEPATITIS B SURFACE ANTIGEN		POSITIVE	POSITIVE		
* HEPATITIS B CORE IGM AB		NONE DETECTED			
* HEPATITIS A IGM ANTIBODY		NONE DETECTED			
* HEPATITIS C ANTIBODY		NON REACTIVE			
* IGA AB		POSITIVE			
* IGG AB		POSITIVE			

Seven weeks 3/8/95	*Eight weeks* 3/15/95	*Seventeen weeks* 5/17/95	*End of treatment* 6/14/95	*Two months later* 8/4/95	*Four months later* 10/27/95	*Fifteen months later* 9/27/96
76	107	91		101	120 H	93
163 H	188 H	188 H		92 H	76 H	135 H
149 H	154 H	100 H		46	25	42
151	135	138		242 H	212 H	222 H

	57			172 H	147 H	159 H
	6.14 L			5.3 H	5.7 H	5.6 H

14.8 H	23.1 H	5.4		2.3 L	3.1 L	3.0 L
3.95 L	3.83 L	4.22 L		4.86	4.47	4.53
12.6 L	11.8 L	13.5 L		15.3	14.5	14.7
41.0	39.2 L	42.2		46.8	44.2	44.5
103.9 H	102.2 H	99.9		96.2	98.8	98.3
31.8	30.8	32.0		31.5	32.3	32.5
30.6 L	30.1 L	32.0		32.7	32.7	33.1
151	109 L	131		184	169	200
79	17	60		26	38	34.4
	18,480 H			598 L	1178 L	1032 L
				150		

Hepatitis BE Antigen	NONE DETECTED	*Hepatitis B DNA QL PCR*	NOT DETECTED			NONE DETECTED
	POSITIVE	NONE DETECTED				NONE DETECTED
Alkaline Phosphatase	134 H	135 H		42	42	
LDH (U/L)	268 H	233		131	115	
AST (U/L)	70 H	51 H		30	22	

THE REST OF THE INTERVIEW OF APRIL 1, 1996
Continued from Chapter Three

Question: Could you talk about what led to your specialization?
Answer: A need to make the world better. This was a field [hepatology] with little or no known cure. I actually wanted to be a Cardiac Surgeon but later diversified.

Question: Are there any interesting experiences or difficult encounters you'd like to discuss?
Answer: There were many things that almost destroyed my medical career, me and my family.

STORY #1:

As a third-year student, I took an advance rotation at a major hospital in Boston. I noticed that three out of four patients died. Here were incompetent older surgeons with terrible techniques performing surgery. On occasion, one of them had alcohol on his breath. I started asking questions and was able to confirm from the operating technicians that these doctors were known to be bad, but were still allowed to perform surgery. I complained to the head of the hospital and was threatened to be kicked out of school if I said anything to anyone. I was told to not be everyone's savior. The head of the hospital did promise to look into the matter and correct the situation. I accepted his promise.

Two years later, an operating technician asked the Boston Globe for help and that exposed the hospital's practices. The operating technician and others who cooperated with the exposure were fired. A book called the "Unkindest Cut" was later written to document the findings. I was quite disappointed that the promise the head of the hospital made to me was not kept. How could anyone be aware of this kind of situation, continue to let these doctors practice and allow innocent people to die? I was quite depressed about the whole situation.

STORY #2:

I was labeled as a troublemaker, not a team player, whistlebower, due to the incident of **STORY #1**. I therefore got my last choice of residency, which was the Veterans Administration (VA) Hospital in Jamaica Plain - Boston, Massachusetts. Most people who went to Harvard Medical School went to Massachusetts General Hosptal, Brigham and Women's, Johns Hopkins hospital or other major/Ivy League hospital - I got the VA, a big referral center.

At the VA, as a blood specialist, I examined a nuclear welder named Adolph Pohopek who was suffering from a rare form of leukemia. Pohopek had worked at the Portsmouth Naval Shipyard in New Hampshire, and asked if radiation exposure at the shipyard might have had anything to do with his leukemia. After examining the situation at the Portsmouth Naval Shipyard, I told Adolph that numerous Portsmouth workers seemed to die unusually young, and that working conditions in the yards were not all they should be. He gave me fifty names of people who had recently worked at Portsmouth.

I found that ten of them were already dead, and I asked the VA for funds to do some follow-up research. The VA turned me down, saying exposures at Portsmouth were too low to have caused any of the deaths. But I persisted. I used my own money, my wife's help, and other resources to send out questionnaires to about forty past and present Portsmouth workers. Within a week the head of the VA's research division in Washington called me, demanding to know who was funding my research and asking for all my correspondence with naval personnel. I asked that the request be put in writing, and never heard from the VA official again.

The questionnaires revealed an alarmingly high rate of leukemia deaths. In mid-November of 1977, I asked The Boston Globe for help. Although the Navy had refused to give me any of its records, I formed an investigative team consisting of my wife, Boston Globe and friends. The Navy refused to release any worker exposure records.

In three months we looked through over 150,000 death certificates by hand, sorting them out by age, date of death, cause of death and if they had worked at the Naval Shipyard. With the help of statistician Dr. Theodore Colton, we assigned a method to determine which former workers, worked with radiation. We asked a series of questions of the families of former workers to confirm that they were exposed to radiation at Portsmouth. We basically asked the Navy four simple questions, one of which was "if I gave you the deceased's name, would you tell me if the person worked with radiation?" The Navy refused to give out radiation records of deceased worker. 1,800 of the 150,000 death certificates identify the Portsmouth Naval Shipyard as the place of employment.

I had to get a disclaimer stating that the work I was doing was on my own and not related to the VA, so as to not get the VA in trouble. I was not and still am not antinuclear. I was just interested in identifying the cause of disease and no one seemed to want to understand nor accept that. Many strange things happened to me at that time that were intended to convince me to stop the investigation, but I ignored them. It's similar to the Karen Silkwood story. Once my study was completed and revealed to the public, I was in the media limelight for a year, giving speeches and being invited to panels to discuss my findings. I felt I had made a difference.

STORY #3:

I got sick with h-pylori (stomach infection) which

causes ulcer. Ibi had the same thing at some point either prior to or during the treatment. My ulcer was bleeding. I don't smoke or drink and could not understand how I got this ulcer. The doctor's suggested treatment was not working. A technician told me about an experimental test for an infection that caused the virus. I researched it and treated myself with antibiotics and it went away. Got the ulcer back later, administered myself another treatment and the ulcer went away permanently. Of course, I reduced my work load after the second treatment and ulcer never came back.

Question: Why did you feel the need to video tape Ibi's consultation session?
Answer: Paranoia and attention to detail. Two of my patients after Ibi told me that with previous doctors, undergoing treatment, no warnings were given to them. I videotaped the session, to communicate the seriousness of the treatment, to emphasize to you how important it is to listen to these things. To make sure that the patient understands that this is a non-standard treatment.

Question: What do you expect from your children?
Answer: It doesn't really matter which field they choose to pursue, as long as they are happy. Mark wanted to be a professional tennis player, so we bought all the best equipment, enrolled him in classes and sent him off to Florida to participate in tournaments and other things which would make him the best tennis player he can be. He later changed his mind. We got rid of the television in the house for about eight months one year because we felt that it didn't help the children grow. We later found out that our children didn't come home and went to friends' houses to watch TV.

Dr. Najarian's Publications

1. Najarian, T. "Journal of American Statistical Society: Comment on Statistics in Epidemiology," November 1983.

2. Najarian, T., Miller, A., Zimelman, A.P., Hong, W.K. "Hematologic Effect of Cis-Platinum-Bleomycin Theraphy," Oncology 38: pp. 195-197, 1981.

3. Najarian, T. "Radiation Induced Myelomatosis," NEJM: p. 1607, June 25, 1981.

4. Castlemen, B. and Najarian, T. "An Unblinded Study of Multiple Myeloma," Chapter 18 of "The Cancer Risks of Low-Level Ionizin Radiation Exposure" prepared by the U.S.G.A.O., E.M.D.M: 1980.

5. Najarian, T. <u>Set For Life? The Insurance Rip-Off and How to Beat It!</u>" SMDN Publishing: 1979.

6. Najarian T. and Castleman, B. "Is Low-Dose Radiation Associated with Myeloma?" NEJM: p. 1278, May 31, 1979.

7. Najarian, T., Miller A., Zimelman, A.P., Hong, W.K. Hematologic Effect of Cis-Platinum-Bleomycin Therapy," Conical Research: p. 390A, April, 1979.

8. Najarian, T., "The Controversy of the Health Effects of Radiation," Technology Review: pp. 74-82, November 1978.

9. Najarian, T. and Colton, T. "Mortality From Leukemia and Cancer in Shipyard Nuclear Workers," The Lancet: pp. 1018-1020, May 13, 1978. This is the original study of Nuclear Workers at the Portsmouth Naval Shipyard done in 1977.

10. Author of a chapter in the book, Power, Pollution and Public Policy, published by the M.I.T. Press, 1971, "Water Quality Improvement in Boston Harbor, p. 242-280. Excerpts from this study were included in Governor Sargent's 1972 Environmental Message to the Legislature, which proposed a $3 Million bond issue to address the sludge disposal problem of the MDC sewer system. This proposal was accepted and active planning to eliminate the problem is now underway.

11. Master's Thesis at M.I.T., "Closed, Continuous-Flow Nutrient Centrifuge for Human Bone Marrow Cultures."

12. Paper presented at the National Junior Science and Humanities Symposium at West Point, New York, 1965, "The Development of an Apparatus for Simultaneous Differential Thermal Analysis, Gas Effluent Analysis and Thermogravimetric Analysis."

Resources

Here are phone numbers to call for more information and/or financial assistance.

Medical Organizations:

American Liver Foundation
1425 Pompton Ave.
Cedar Grove, NJ 07009
Phone: 1-800-223-0179

Center for Disease Control (CDC) Hepatitis Hotline
Phone: (404) 332-4555

Office for the Study of Unconventional Medical Practices
National Institute of Health
Building 31, Room 2B25
Bethesda, MD 20892
Phone: (301) 496-7498

National Digestive Diseases Information Clearinghouse
2 Information Way
Bethesda, MD 20892-3570
Phone: (301) 654-3810

Phamaceutical Assistance

Schering U.S. Committment to Care Program
This program provides reimbursement assistance, video and other educational materials.
1-800-521-7157

Schering Canada has an 800 number to learn more about hepatitis, and a second number to help find financial assistance to receive Interferon.

Information for Patients
1-800-363-3422
code 2121

Information for Physicians
1-800-463-4636
code 437

Information regarding financial assistance
1-800-363-3422,
extension 2000

Hepatitis Network and Referral Service

These organizations provide telephone support and some do have supports group. They all serve as referal centers and can direct you to liver specialists in your area. Please take note of its groups focus. Their names usually states their niche. If it does not, it means one can get assistance with any type of Hepatitis. For example, the American Liver Foundation has a wealth of information about all types of Hepatitis.

Please note that some of these organizations are in the process of developing web pages and setting up satelite sites, no final information is available at this time.

United States

American Liver Foundation, Rocky Mountain Chapter
Hepatitis B and Pediatric Focus
Rocky Mountain, Colorado
Phone: 1-888-OK-LIVER
President: Lee Gerstner

American Liver Foundation
1425 Pompton Avenue
Cedar Grove, NJ 07009-1000
Phone: 1-800-GO-LIVER, 201-256-2550
fax: 201-256-3214
President: Alan P. Brownstein

The HepConnection, Colorado Hepatitis C Network and Support System
For more information contact Ann Jesse:
Phone: (303) 393-9395
President: Ann Jesse

Hepatitis Foundation International
30 Sunrise Terrace
Cedar Grove, NJ 07009
Phone: (201) 239-1035, 1-800-891-0707
fax: (201) 857-5044
President: Thelma King Thiel

The Hepatitis C Foundation
1502 Russett Drive
Warminster, PA 18972
Phone: (215) 672-2606
e-mail: HEPATITIS_C_FOUNDATION@msn.com

Alaska (Anchorage) Hepatitis Support Group
Phone: (907) 562-9150
e-mail: clotho@corcom.com

Indianapolis, Indiana HCV Support Group
Phone: (317) 879-6168

United Liver Association
11646 West Pico Blvd.
Los Angeles, CA 90064
Phone: (310) 914-8252

Hepatitis Education Project
P.O. Box 95162
Seattle, WA 98145
Phone: (206) 447-8136
e-mail: graham@phoenix.artsci.washington.edu

Eastside Hepatitis Education Project
Eastside Group Health Hospital
Redmond, Washington
Phone: (206) 562-0980

Liver Center at St. Francis Medical Center
St. Francis Hospital
228 Liliha Street, MOB 200
Honolulu, Hawaii 96817
3rd Wednesday of every month from 7:00 PM to 9:00 PM
Phone: (808) 547-6995

Iowa Hepatitis Educational Project & Support
Phone: (319) 351-7860
e-mail: webbsite@inav.net
President: Elizabeth Fell-Webb

AUSTRALIA

Hepatitis C Council of NSW
P.O. Box 432
Darlinghurst, NSW 2010
Info/support phone: (02) 1-800-803 990, Sydney callers should use (02) 9332-1599
Administration phone: or (02) 9332-1853
Fax: (02) 9332-1730
Office address:
Level 2/345 Crown Street
Surry Hills, NSW 2010
email: 100357.263@compuserve.com
Executive Officer: Stuart Loveday
Senior Project Officer: Paul Harvey
President: Cheryl Burman

The Hepatitis C Foundation (VIC) Inc.
Fairfield Hospital
Yarra Bend Road
Fairfield
Phone: Melbourne (03) 280 2317

The Hepatitis C Council of Queensland
P.O. Box 179
Albert Street

Brisbane, Queensland, Australia
Info/support line: (07) 3229 3767
Queensland FreeCall: 1800 648 491
Administration: (07) 3229 9238
Fax: (07) 3229 9305
e-mail: hepcq@powerup.com.au
Queensland Intravenous AIDS Association/
Hepatitis C Support (QuIVAA)
93 Brunswick Street, Fortitude Valley
Brisbane 4006, Queensland, Australia
Phone: 07-32 52 53 90
Fax: 07-32 52 53 92
E-mail: quivaa@powerup.com.au
Lecture/support group meetings are held on the last Thursday of every month.
Co-ordinator: Mr Jeff Ward

The Macfarlane Burnet Centre for Medical Research
PO Box 254, Fairfield
Victoria 3078
AUSTRALIA
Phone: (+61 3) 9282 2169
Fax: (+61 3) 9482 3123
email: crofts@burnet.mbcmr.unimelb.edu.au

CANADA

Canadian Liver Foundation
365 Bloor Street East, Suite 200
Toronto, Ontario M4W 3L4
Phone: (416) 964-1953
Toll-free within Canada only: 1-800-563-5483
Fax: (416) 964-0024
email addresses:
Communications/Public Relations:
smith@liver.ca or porchuk@liver.ca
Patient Information:
potkonjak@liver.ca or lizee@liver.ca
President: Ms. Lorraine Smith

Hepatitis C Survivors Society
383 Huron Street
Toronto, Ontario, Canada M5S 2G5
Toll-free within Canada only: 1-800-652-HEPC
phone: (416) 979-5855
fax: (416) 979-5856

BTV Hepatitis "C" Foundation
P.O. Box 21040
Penticton, B.C. V2A 8K8
phone: (604) 490-9054
fax: (604) 490-0620
e-mail: Peter Gibbenhuck at pgibbenh@mail.awinc.com

UNITED KINGDOM

The British Liver Trust
Phone: 01473 276326

Royal Free Hospital Liver Patients' Support Group (London)
Phone: 0171 794 0500 ext 4909
President: Sheila Cooper

St Mary's Liver Patients' Support Group (London)
Phone: 0181 458 7009
President: Eugenia Toon

URUGUAY

Grupo C
c/o Centro Anglicano de Solidaridad y Ayuda
Reconquista 625
Montevideo, Uruguay
telefax: (02) 955 419
e-mail: freno@chasque.apc.org

INDEX

This index is intended to highlight key items.

Notes

Notes

ORDER FORM

The Cure of Chronic Hepatitis B, One Man's Cure, One Family's Experience

A donation from each sale will be made to the Corporate & Children's Hepatitis Foundation started by IROK Solutions Inc.

1 book		@ $19.95	
2 - 4 books	______	@ $18.95 each	= $__________
5 - 9 books	______	@ $17.95 each	= $__________
10 - 24 books	______	@ $16.95 each	= $__________
25 and over	______	@ $15.95 each	= $__________

Price is in United States dollar currency.

WITHIN U.S. SHIPPING IS $3.95 FOR FIRST BOOK, $2.95 PER ADDITIONAL BOOKS.
No. of books ____ - 1 = _____ x $2.95 = ______ + $3.95 = $_________

TOTAL COST = COST OF BOOK(S)_______ + SHIPPING ______ = $_________

FOUR WAYS TO ORDER

FAX ORDERS: Toll Free 1-888-IROKSOL (1-888-476-5765)

TELEPHONE ORDERS: Call Toll Free 1-888-IROKSOL

ORDER THRU THE INTERNET:
http://www.bookzone.com/bookzone/10000853.html

MAIL ORDERS: IROK Solutions Inc., 1770 Mass Ave, Suite 134
Cambridge, MA 02140, U.S.A.

☐ CHECK ENCLOSED ☐ VISA ☐ MasterCard

ACCOUNT NUMBER______________________________ EXP. DATE___________

SIGNATURE____

ORDER FORM

The Cure of Chronic Hepatitis B, One Man's Cure, One Family's Experience

A donation from each sale will be made to the Corporate & Children's Hepatitis Foundation started by IROK Solutions Inc.

1 book		@ $19.95	
2 - 4 books	______	@ $18.95 each	= $__________
5 - 9 books	______	@ $17.95 each	= $__________
10 - 24 books	______	@ $16.95 each	= $__________
25 and over	______	@ $15.95 each	= $__________

Price is in United States dollar currency.

WITHIN U.S. SHIPPING IS $3.95 FOR FIRST BOOK, $2.95 PER ADDITIONAL BOOKS.
No. of books ____ - 1 = _____ x $2.95 = ______ + $3.95 = $_________

TOTAL COST = COST OF BOOK(S)_______ + SHIPPING ______ = $_________

FOUR WAYS TO ORDER

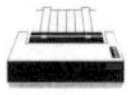

FAX ORDERS: Toll Free 1-888-IROKSOL (1-888-476-5765)

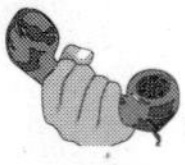

TELEPHONE ORDERS: Call Toll Free 1-888-IROKSOL

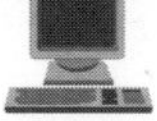

ORDER THRU THE INTERNET:
http://www.bookzone.com/bookzone/10000853.html

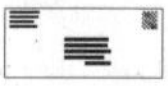

MAIL ORDERS: IROK Solutions Inc., 1770 Mass Ave, Suite 134
Cambridge, MA 02140, U.S.A.

☐ CHECK ENCLOSED ☐ VISA ☐ MasterCard

ACCOUNT NUMBER______________________________ EXP. DATE___________

SIGNATURE____